Humanizing Addiction Practice

Antoine Douaihy · H. Patrick Driscoll

Humanizing Addiction Practice

Blending Science and Personal Transformation

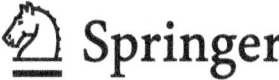

Antoine Douaihy
Western Psychiatric Institute and Clinic
University of Pittsburgh School of Medicine
Pittsburgh, PA
USA

H. Patrick Driscoll
Western Psychiatric Institute and Clinic
University of Pittsburgh School of Medicine
Pittsburgh, PA
USA

ISBN 978-3-319-91004-8   ISBN 978-3-319-91005-5 (eBook)
https://doi.org/10.1007/978-3-319-91005-5

Library of Congress Control Number: 2018944121

© Springer International Publishing AG, part of Springer Nature 2018
This work is subject to copyright. All rights are reserved by the Publisher, whether the whole or part of the material is concerned, specifically the rights of translation, reprinting, reuse of illustrations, recitation, broadcasting, reproduction on microfilms or in any other physical way, and transmission or information storage and retrieval, electronic adaptation, computer software, or by similar or dissimilar methodology now known or hereafter developed.
The use of general descriptive names, registered names, trademarks, service marks, etc. in this publication does not imply, even in the absence of a specific statement, that such names are exempt from the relevant protective laws and regulations and therefore free for general use.
The publisher, the authors and the editors are safe to assume that the advice and information in this book are believed to be true and accurate at the date of publication. Neither the publisher nor the authors or the editors give a warranty, express or implied, with respect to the material contained herein or for any errors or omissions that may have been made. The publisher remains neutral with regard to jurisdictional claims in published maps and institutional affiliations.

Printed on acid-free paper

This Springer imprint is published by the registered company Springer International Publishing AG part of Springer Nature
The registered company address is: Gewerbestrasse 11, 6330 Cham, Switzerland

To Neil Capretto whose gentle spirit, empathy, generosity, and compassion healed innumerable lives. R.I.P., Neil: you are already missed.
—Antoine Douaihy

To the "Prof," Harrison J. Pemberton, who blended empathy and understanding into the kind of pedagogy that has become for me the inspiration for every teaching (and learning) moment that I've been a part of since he helped me decide on medicine and psychiatry many years ago.
—H. Patrick Driscoll

Epigraph

"I find I am at my best when I can let the flow of my experience carry me...."

—Carl Rogers

Foreword 1

Stories and science. As relational creatures, we are enthralled and inspired by stories of the experiences and adventures of our fellow travelers in life. As rational creatures, we are captivated and intrigued by scientific findings that provide insight into ourselves and our world. This book speaks to both these aspects of our personhood. It contains personal stories and scientific advances that address the challenges faced by individuals dealing with addiction and by therapists seeking to help them. The lead author, Antoine Douaihy, is a consummate and richly experienced physician-scientist-teacher of addiction medicine. He is ably assisted by a mentee and colleague, H. Patrick Driscoll, who brings the important perspectives of one newer to the field. Together, they have crafted a very readable and readily accessible summary of what we currently understand about the nature of addiction, and thoughtful and transparent travel logs of those who are on the journey to recovery and of those who are helping them. I highly recommend it to anyone who seeks to advance their abilities to understand and help those dealing with addiction.

David A. Lewis, MD
Department of Psychiatry and Neuroscience
University of Pittsburgh, School of Medicine
Pittsburgh, PA
USA

Foreword 2

This is an informative, insightful, and inspiring book that incorporates science, the wisdom of many great thinkers, the experiences of individuals and family members in recovery, and reflections of the authors' struggles and successes as addiction psychiatrists. Healthcare professionals and others will find many lessons from Dr. Douaihy's extensive knowledge, clinical savvy, and personal insights about his work with patients and families who live with addiction and, in many cases, co-existing psychiatric and medical disorders. He educates the reader about the major findings from science and debunks some of the awful, negative myths about addiction, its treatment, and recovery. The reader learns that there is hope for recovery and that practitioners can make a significant impact if they overcome their personal biases and negative reactions to individuals suffering from an addiction.

Numerous clinical stories evidence the emotional and spiritual pain, numerous problems and struggles of patients and families affected by addiction, as well as their growth, resiliency, and recovery. Despite the challenges posed by these complex stories, Antoine shows that professionals can make a significant impact if they are empathic, connect and "be with" patients by entering their world, and work collaboratively in an accepting and nonjudgmental manner. He conveys clearly that his best teachers are his patients and their families. The book shows how he provides hope to patients and family members who often feel despair and hopelessness, and he shares meaningfully in their healing journey.

Antoine shows how he successfully blends the "art" of healing as a psychiatrist with the "science" of evidenced-based interventions based on clinical trials. He espouses the importance of religion and spirituality in addiction recovery for many patients, shows there are many pathways to recovery, and understands the pain and heartache of families and the need to consider the impact of addiction on them and engage them in treatment and recovery. He conveys the important role of mutual support programs for individuals with addiction and family members. He understands how family systems impact patients and how patients impact the family system by focusing on much more than symptoms or behaviors associated with an addiction.

One of the many strengths of this book is Antoine's self-disclosure about his struggles in practice. Anyone who knows him would describe him as one of the most knowledgeable, skillful, and effective practitioners they have ever met. Yet, he does a remarkable job exposing his vulnerabilities, self-doubt, failures and weaknesses as a psychiatrist, and feelings of anger and disappointment at patients. His "humanism" shines through, making this book more appealing and readable.

I have had the honor of meeting and working with many of the best thinkers (researchers, clinicians, both) about addiction in our country from the top universities and health institutes. I can say that very few are as knowledgeable and skillful as Antoine in clinical care, teaching, and mentoring, and in sharing their experiences, facing their limitations, and becoming a more compassionate caregiver. Antoine mentors professionals from numerous disciplines and is an exceptional teacher who is well regarded and respected. I read many self-reflective statements about clinical experiences of those he has mentored in clinical settings. All were rich with self-disclosure of personal flaws, worries, and limitations. Yet, all showed tremendous personal and professional growth in their ability to help a clinical population often judged negatively by practitioners. I truly believe this book will educate and inspire readers.

Dennis C. Daley, PhD
Department of Psychiatry
University of Pittsburgh Medical Center
Pittsburgh, PA
USA

Humanizing Addiction Practice

How does one meld scientific expertise with the process of becoming an empathic patient-centered healer? Drs. Douaihy and Driscoll offer an engaging story of their own professional development, describing patient encounters that helped to shape their humane approach to the practice of science-based addiction medicine. Evident throughout the book is their contagious appreciation of the privilege of witnessing firsthand so many journeys of recovery.

William R. Miller, PhD
Emeritus Distinguished Professor
of Psychology and Psychiatry,
University of New Mexico,
Albuquerque, NM
USA

Preface

Imagine being labeled by society as a self-indulgent, morally corrupt, pathological liar. Not uncommonly, the popular media portrays individuals struggling with addiction in these disparaging terms. Even the healthcare practitioners charged with treating these individuals are not immune and can either consciously or unwittingly reflect these underlying judgments in their interactions. Individuals with addictions—ever adept at anticipating and reading the reactions of others—not only register these rejections but also internalize the belief that they are simply no good. This diminishing of the individual with addiction complicates the recovery process and impedes self-discovery not only for those struggling but, ironically, also for those providing care. These subtle attitudes can undermine their recovery journey as well as our partnership with them along the way.

Unfortunately, negative attitudes towards people suffering from addiction have spawned treatment approaches that engender distrust of the healthcare system and of its practitioners. These attitudes either dissuade individuals from seeking care altogether or negatively impact the therapeutic process. Particularly corrosive are the beliefs that persons with addictions deserve what they get, have brought on their own problems, lack the capacity to change, or do not want to change. Skepticism about a person's desire for or likelihood of change further complicates the therapeutic process and can impair the ever-important sense of hope, for patients and practitioners alike. Frustrated caregivers can resort to blaming their patients for not changing or not changing fast enough. They may adopt beliefs that treatment will not work unless the patient is ready and motivated to change. Statements such as "come back when you're motivated" and/or "when you hit rock bottom" ensue. These statements, however, serve to further impair the therapeutic relationship, perpetuate mistrust, and delay recovery. In the end, the belief one has about addiction, whom it affects, and how likely an individual struggling with it is to change will significantly impact treatment outcomes. In ways we as caregivers may not always appreciate, these beliefs can also undermine our sense of ourselves as caring professionals. So, while the struggle with addiction can degenerate meaning in a person's life, recovery offers the possibility of rediscovering what is lost. This search for meaning is not unique to persons with addictions. It also extends to the people who love them, as well as the individuals who seek to work with them in the recovery process.

In recently reflecting on how I have evolved as a person and an addiction psychiatrist, I found myself and my career totally consumed and devastated by America's deadly opioid public health crisis. I have been losing patients, seeing their families torn apart, and their communities decimated. As I was rethinking my practice and advocacy work, I went through an existential career crisis which ultimately strengthened my ethical and moral values, and my ability to manage uncertainty, and helped me maintain intellectual and emotional humility. I realized, more than ever before, that I must strive to integrate science and humanism, approaching addiction from a socio-cultural perspective, conceptualizing it as fueled by the poor sense of community and connectedness. I started shifting my practice to emphasize, first and foremost, on helping patients and their families establish growth-fostering relationships and values. I wanted to be part of their reclaiming their dignity and purpose in life.

My patients, quite simply, have provided me with courage and self-understanding. I have been moved and inspired by them in ways I could not have imagined. To pay homage to them I hold nothing back and instead share my innermost experiences—my successes, failures, triumphs, and mistakes. And there have been mistakes. Major mistakes. I have grown from them. I am committed to assisting those who come after me to know what matters, what works, and what does not. I am thankful for the meaning my work has brought me, and through this book I try to candidly portray my experiences and path.

I believe that the process of self-understanding is a fundamental aspect of medical education and medical practice. I have realized through working with medical trainees, physicians, researchers, and educators that this process is seldom recognized, understood, or nurtured, and even less often respected. Only after I allowed the boundary between my professional self and my personal self to blur was I able to garner true gratification and fulfillment in my career and, ironically, in my life. It is the personal sharing of my patients' struggles that has provided me meaning, a meaning I hope is well reflected on the pages that follow.

Through a lifelong commitment to introspection, I have often asked myself: What is compelling about sharing the most challenging, emotionally charged aspects of my addiction practice? How can I help the next generation of practitioners learn from my clinical life? I am hopeful you will be able to walk with me through this journey of finding answers and, perhaps more importantly, asking new questions.

This book is about my professional journey. I have spent my entire career drafting it. It is about healing addiction and is as much about the ways in which my patients have changed me as it is about my helping them. I reflect upon the lessons I have learned from my patients, lessons that were available nowhere else. It is an account of the years of interactions I have had with my patients and their families and the way these interactions have contributed more to my professional identity and growth than my schooling and training. To help my patients, I have been privileged to share and experience their suffering, all while simultaneously striving to maintain the ever-elusive level of separateness necessary to be clinically effective.

These experiences have hurt me, scarred me, pushed me, invigorated me, and changed me. They have given my life meaning. Without these experiences, I would not be the person I am, and this book could not be written. Each person has shaped my views of addiction, of helping, of treatment, and of so much more. Throughout the book, I make every effort to capture the essence of my journey by reflecting on my vulnerabilities, mistakes, doubts, fears, prejudices, and constant search for a therapeutic emotional connection beyond the standards of technical competence.

It was during my years of training and practice in addiction as I wondered about how to better appreciate integrating scientific and humanistic elements in the therapeutic work that this book took shape. I have been monitoring myself to avoid slipping into a position of arrogance, that of believing I know best. It is through this lens of humanity embedded in empirical evidence that I aspire to share my experiences and those of others. These stories are a memorialization of how humanity, personhood, and clinical acumen are together indispensable if one is to effect real change and transformation. My patients taught me to be open-minded, flexible, pragmatic, less focused on "disease" and "morality," and more on a better understanding of the complexity of human suffering. At the same time, they taught me how to practice evidence-based medicine and apply relevant clinical science to their unique struggles, values, and personal wishes. Healthcare practitioners cannot simply rely on scientific curiosity, mastery of medical knowledge, and an impersonal set of technical skills to make a difference. They must communicate, connect, hurt, and feel. All of this will help them understand their patients, their patients' suffering, and most importantly, themselves. Only when these things coalesce will they be effective healers.

I describe here how I discovered, developed, and grew in my career in addiction psychiatry and how I keep hope that my patients will improve and become themselves. It is about my own self-growth and about forging a sense of values for living well and being fulfilled with my work. As such, this is a *personal* book.

This book is written in the *spirit* of collaborative exploration with Dr. Driscoll (HPD), a former trainee of mine and a master of the written clinical word, who will give my professional experiences an exceptional clarity by allowing me to open my heart to him and by offering stimulating perspectives from his own career development. HPD shares that:

> "*I could only have fulfillment in my professional work by being personally open to the emotions and struggles that the patient encounters aroused in me. It was only by taking responsibility for these thoughts and feelings as issues of my own that I could feel freer to engage and be with the patient without feeling stymied or fettered by the biases and prejudices that make addiction work less meaningful. I also learned to use lessons from my trainings in ways that I had not anticipated: I did not learn medical knowledge that could be used to educate others; I had to repurpose the content of what I learned so that I could share it in a way consistent with receiving the patient as a whole person rather than just an "utterer of symptoms and a displayer of signs."*

Though names, case materials, and clinical details of individual patients have been altered, the universal impact of their disclosures and experiences endure.

Wherever appropriate, permission has been requested and kindly granted. It is my hope that others learn from these clinical stories, too, and be inspired. They certainly offered me many enlightening lessons that built the foundation for my identity as an addiction psychiatrist.

A few words about language. Throughout the book, I have sought to use *addiction (or person with an addiction)* as the most generic term for substance use disorders as well as other addictive behaviors and disorders. My fundamental goal was to avoid jargon, as well as pejorative and judgmental terms and labels, which also forced me to think more humanistically and scientifically about the complex issues of addictive behaviors.

What can the reader expect to learn by immersion in this voyage of self-discovery through sharing clinical experiences in addiction settings? I believe a great deal. Sharing my personal experiences through emotional writing and discussing what transpires in difficult clinical encounters made me focus better on how best to help my most challenging patients and facilitated my growth as a *healer*. I offer you an invitation to draw on the challenges and struggles I describe to create learning experiences for your own practice.

Within this book are key lessons for healthcare professionals: lessons learned from decades of therapeutic experiences, as well as recommendations about how to use these lessons for emotional growth over the course of a career. The primary audience for this book consists of healers of *all* kinds: physicians, social workers, nurse practitioners, case managers, patient navigators, clinical and health psychologists, physician assistants, pharmacists, members of clergy, counselors, and peers. Medical trainees (students/residents/fellows) who are involved in everyday clinical care in almost every branch of medicine and in diverse healthcare settings (and who often underestimate their ability to foster change in patients) as well as educators and students in the respective aforementioned domains also will benefit from this book.

Recommended Readings

1. Douaihy A, Kelly TM, Gold MA. Motivational interviewing: a guide for medical trainees. New York: Oxford University Press; 2015.
2. Miller WR. Lovingkindness: realizing and practicing your true self. Eugene, OR: Cascade Books; 2017.
3. Brendel DH. Healing psychiatry, bridging the science/humanism divide. Cambridge, MA: The MIT Press; 2006.

Pittsburgh, PA, USA Antoine Douaihy, MD
Pittsburgh, PA, USA H. Patrick Driscoll, MD, MSc

Prologue

The prologue introduces the reader to the importance of understanding addiction and the impact of negative and prejudiced attitudes towards people who struggle with addiction and links that with the author's own "voice," experiences, journey, transformation, and the formation of his identity as an addiction psychiatrist. It invites the reader to treat addiction using a science-based approach integrated within a humanistic framework.

Acknowledgments

I want to express my regard and deep appreciation to my friend, colleague, and coauthor Patrick Driscoll, the virtuoso of spoken word. Your tactful insight, compassion, humility, unwavering support, and, above all, exceptional ability to take my private thoughts and make them come eloquently to fruition on paper will be forever cherished. Thank you for your unique perspectives and your unceasing faith in my work; I will forever be grateful. Special gratitude is owed to Dennis Daley, whose mentorship, unwavering intellectual and emotional support contributed to this work. I wish to acknowledge my indebtedness to my former mentors during my residency training and career, and especially Ihsan Salloum and Frank Ghinassi, for their commitment to my professional and personal growth. This book was made possible because of the work and influence of pioneers in the field of addiction and motivational interviewing: Bill Miller, Steve Rollnick, Alan Marlatt, and Dennis Daley, who guided my thinking, instilled in me a powerful understanding of humanity, and made me believe in the healing power of therapeutic work. A special thanks to David Lewis: I am inspired by his leadership, wisdom, and humility. I'm deeply indebted to my colleagues at Western Psychiatric Institute and Clinic, the University of Pittsburgh Medical Center, and the University of Pittsburgh School of Medicine for providing an empathic and stimulating milieu in which to work. Many people have supported me, in one way or another, in the writing of the book, and I owe special thanks particularly to Cindy Hurney, Dorothy Sandstrom, Leslie Sullivan, and Amy Shanahan. I also wish to express my gratitude to Rachel Levine, Cele Fichter-DeSando, Joan Ward, Kevork Wannissian, Daniel Cohen, Linda Frank, Mike Flaherty, Mike Lynch, and Amy and Neil Capretto for their encouragement and the wisdom of their insight and experiences. I have been privileged to learn and contribute to the learning experiences of medical trainees and other healthcare practitioners who value science and empathy. I wish to acknowledge my indebtedness to the following individuals who all contributed to the experiences and perspectives in this book: John Eisnman, Annie Lu, Jen Forsyth, Isaac Petersen, Erin Smith, Brittany Atuahene, Emilie Transue, Lauren Goldshen, Jennifer Darby, M. Usama Hindiyeh, Alexandra Sansosti, Shriya Kaneriya, and Gil Hoftman. I must extend my utmost respect and gratitude to my patients and their families, who taught me innumerable lessons in courage, hope, tolerance, empathy, humility, and compassion. I cannot say enough to thank my parents, family, and friends for their love and support. Finally, this manuscript could not have been completed without the help and wonderful support of Elizabeth Corra and Richard Lansing of Springer Nature.

Antoine Douaihy, MD

Thank you to Antoine Douaihy for being a friend, a teacher, and an inspiration in every clinical moment during which first I have struggled and then asked, "What would Antoine do?" Those moments have formed the nucleus of the experience that has gone into this book. If the best therapy amounts to a kind of spoken poetry within which a mind may dwell, then trying to emulate Antoine's example of caring and teaching has been a way of making this work a home. I did not always think it possible to find such a meaningful place to live. I am also deeply grateful to "the Prof," Harrison J. Pemberton, who first made me aware of such a life of the mind but who passed on before he could see the words in this book that he inspired. I still don't know if it was knowing him or being known by him that was so transformative. I would like to thank my family, especially my parents, John and Anne Driscoll, for their love and support at every stage of the way. Theirs were acts and examples of selfless devotion and sacrifice to make possible so many opportunities for growing and learning. I also want to mention my nephews and nieces—Michael, Molly, Alexander, Quinn, Margaret, and Frances—for being so spurringly present in my thoughts over the years. I am also grateful to Jessica Packer, Colleen Carney, Jeff McCurry, Paula Moreci, Michael Pauly, Jonathan Reese, and Vikrant Rachakonda for sharing each of their minds (and stories) in such helpful and enriching ways. Michael gave me some of the best advice I received in medical school: "You should do a rotation with Antoine Douaihy on the dual diagnosis unit before you leave Pittsburgh," he told me in our final year. "He's an insightful guy." So I did. I have been here collaborating with him ever since. Thank you to Robert M. Brosh, Kreg Mendus, and Charles F. Reynolds for early life and career mentorship. I am also indebted to all my colleagues and trainees at Western Psychiatric Institute and Clinic, at the Pittsburgh Psychoanalytic Center, and throughout the University of Pittsburgh School of Medicine for their support and teaching. Finally, thank you to everyone who allowed me to walk with them through some part of their lives and tolerated some of the most intimate questions about their vulnerabilities, hopes, and dreams. On the wards or in the consulting room, I am grateful for the experiences that patients have allowed me to have with them. These moments have made for the most fulfilling professional experience I could have imagined at this early point in my career.

H. Patrick Driscoll, MD, MSc

Contents

Part I On Relationships, Empathy, Healing, and Growth

1 Building a Mindset for Healing 3
　References 18

2 Cultivating Empathy and Emotional Openness in Practice 21
　References 28

3 Learning and Growing from Unpredictable Encounters 31
　References 42

Part II On Integrating Science and Humanistic Practice

4 Scientific Foundations for Addiction Practice 45
　Introduction 45
　Historical Context and Theoretical Models of Addiction 46
　Where Is the Origin of Social Stigma and Pessimism? 47
　Reasons for Optimism and Hope: Key Issues
　　in Treatment Effectiveness 52
　The Effect of the Therapist in Addiction Treatment:
　　Relationship Matters 53
　Motivational Interviewing: My Path towards Clinical
　　and Personal Transformation 54
　Relapse Prevention 58
　Pharmacological Treatments 59
　Seven Robust Scientific Findings Informing Clinical Practices 60
　References 61

5 Working with Family and Significant Others 65
　Introduction 65
　Myths About Families and Addiction 66
　Impact of Substance Use Disorders on Family and Children 67

Typical Concerns of Family Members About Co-Occurring Disorders	70
Family-Based Interventions: What Works?	71
References	74

6 Spirituality, Religion, and Mutual Support Programs ... 77
Introduction ... 77
Spirituality and Religion ... 78
    Spiritual and Religious Treatments for Addiction ... 78
    Practical Considerations for Healthcare Practitioners
    About Spirituality and Addiction ... 79
Mutual Support Programs ... 80
    The Varieties of Mutual Support Programs ... 80
    12-Step Programs ... 81
Reflections from Clinical Practice ... 85
References ... 87

Part III On Teaching, Learning, and Meaning

7 Trainees' Reflections on Clinical and Personal Growth ... 93
Introduction ... 93
Learning to Treat Addictions by Embracing the Spirit of MI:
Jen Forsyth, 2016 ... 94
Humanizing Practice Through MI as a Means of Clinical
and Personal Transformation: Isaac Petersen, 2016 ... 95
First Experience Learning to Work Therapeutically
Using MI as a Way of Walking In-Step with the Patient:
Erin Smith, 2012 ... 96
Humanistic Approach Using MI as a Vehicle for Advocacy
for Patients: Brittany Atuahene, 2017 ... 97
Humanistic Approach as Means of Empathic Connection
Between Different Walks of Life: Emilie Transue, 2017 ... 98
MI as a Way to Replenish One's Personal (and Clinical!) Spirit:
Lauren Goldshen, 2017 ... 99
Humanistic Practice as Means to Self-Discovery: Jennifer Darby, 2017 ... 100
Person-Centered Approach as Supplement to Treating Serious
Chronic Illnesses and Understanding the True Meaning
of Empathy: M. Usama Hindiyeh, 2017 ... 101
Humanistic Practice as a Treatment for the Trainee's Soul ... 102
    Alexandra Sansosti, 2017 ... 102
    Shriya Kaneriya, 2017 ... 104
    Gil Hoftman, 2017 ... 106
    H. Patrick Driscoll, 2018 ... 108
Conclusion ... 110
Recommended Readings ... 110

Epilogue ... 111

Index ... 115

About the Authors

Antoine Douaihy, MD is professor of psychiatry and medicine at the University of Pittsburgh School of Medicine. He also serves as the senior academic director of Addiction Medicine Services and director of the Addiction Psychiatry Fellowship at Western Psychiatric Institute and Clinic (WPIC) of the University of Pittsburgh Medical Center. His addiction practice focuses mostly on providing care for patients and families on the dual diagnosis unit at WPIC. He has established his career on patient care/advocacy, education, training, and research in the areas of motivational interviewing, substance use disorders, and HIV/AIDS. In recognition for his dedication to patient care, education, and training, Dr. Douaihy has been the recipient of multiple awards, including the Leonard Tow Humanism in Medicine Award and the Charles Watson Teaching Award, recognizing him for the qualities of a masterful clinician, academician, caretaker of his patients, educator, mentor, and contributor to the medical school community and the community at large.

H. Patrick Driscoll, MD, MSc is clinical assistant professor of child and adolescent psychiatry at the University of Pittsburgh Medical Center and candidate at the Pittsburgh Psychoanalytic Center. In addition to his psychiatric research background and providing care to patients and families on the inpatient addiction and child and adolescent units, his private practice focuses on helping people throughout the life cycle (and their loved ones) through motivationally based, behavioral, and insight-oriented treatments often in combination with psychopharmacologic interventions. He also serves on the board of the Clinic Without Walls, a low fee psychodynamic psychotherapy clinic. His career has focused on teaching and supervising medical trainees at all levels in motivational interviewing, dialectical behavioral therapy, family interventions, combined medication and psychotherapeutic treatment, and psychodynamic and psychoanalytic psychotherapies. In recognition of his passion for education and dedication to patient care, Dr. Driscoll has received numerous teaching awards from medical students, residents, and fellows. In 2015, he received the Clerkship Preceptor of the Year Award from the University of Pittsburgh School of Medicine, which recognized him for outstanding achievements in educating future physicians.

Part I
On Relationships, Empathy, Healing, and Growth

"Growth occurs when individuals confront problems, struggle to master them, and through that struggle develop new aspects of their skills, capacities, views about life."

—Carl Rogers: A Way of Being, 1995: 134.

Part I describes my career journey, exploring the process of becoming an empathic patient-centered healer. To lay this groundwork, it weaves my discovery of foundational psychotherapeutic approaches and the all-important clinical stories that have shaped my identity. I will show how the experiences I shared with my patients cultivated empathic attunement, compassion, and cognitive and emotional flexibility. Part I goes on to examine what leads to misunderstanding of patients' suffering and also challenges the traditional assumptions that emotional detachment provides more objectivity. I argue instead for *more* connectedness, and I will attempt to show how this connection structures and deepens our therapeutic influence as healers. I have discovered that it is this connection that puts the humanistic spirit into action.

Chapter 1
Building a Mindset for Healing

> *"The meeting of two personalities is like the contact of two chemical substances: if there is any reaction, both are transformed."*
>
> —Carl Jung: Modern Man in Search of a Soul, 1955

I started to write this book because in the heart of every clinical experience I had with a patient there is a unique story. To learn this story means to sit and share with the patient a seat on a roller coaster of complex emotions, suffering, expectations, missteps, intimate moments both mundane and divine, culminating in hope, change, transformation, and healing. Throughout my writing, I seek a tone of voice that binds the scientific with the humanistic and the personal as integral aspects of the healing process. When I think *patient encounter*, I imagine not only a helping relationship but also, and more importantly, a healing relationship. Walant [1] described the powerful mutual impact of the connection between two separate beings in an encounter: "feel[ing] themselves into the other."

In medical school, my first exposures to clinical realities highlighted my total naiveté about the therapeutic work. As I recall, I knew almost nothing about substance use disorders and I was unfamiliar with the conceptual models of addiction, treatment approaches, and their effectiveness. Furthermore, I had received barely any training related to alcohol and drug problems. Thinking back, I cannot even remember the topic of substance use disorders being reviewed in detail either in the mainstream courses in medical school nor in my psychiatry residency program. My attitude was neutral: I thought maybe substance issues were not a major problem that I would encounter much in my professional life, and I wondered if perhaps they would be addressed only by the specialists in the field of addiction.

My interest in and passion for addiction work started coincidentally when I was assigned my first mentor, who is an addiction psychiatrist, in my first year of residency training back in 1992. He loved the field and ignited in me a powerful curiosity about discovering what it is like to be working with people with substance use disorders. I felt a natural sense of belonging with something, finding out that it was the pursuit of a career in addiction. It was then that I started actively seeking clinical opportunities that exposed me more to working with individuals with addictions. A totally immersive experience! Reaching out to my mentor for guidance on what to read and where to find this literature, he recommended three main volumes: *Motivational Interviewing: Preparing People to Change Addictive Behavior* by William R. Miller and Stephen Rollnick (1991) [2], *Alcoholics Anonymous: The Story of How More than One Hundred Men Have Recovered from Alcoholism* by Bill Wilson (1939) [3], and *Relapse Prevention: Maintenance Strategies in the Treatment of Addictive Behaviors* edited by G. Alan Marlatt and Judith R. Gordon (1985) [4]. I was somewhat confused and overwhelmed: So much to know and learn about addictive behaviors and addictions! The major challenges that I started facing were related to synthesizing the most current scientific knowledge regarding substance use disorders and how to make use of it. Tapping into the research, I was fascinated by the tremendous number of studies and findings that were published and at the same time disturbed by the significant delay in the diffusion of innovative and effective research into clinical practices and programs. History has shown us for decades that healthcare practitioners, systems of care, supervision, and training programs as well as policymakers have adopted practices and policies that were rarely informed by science. Change takes time, and addressing the research-to-treatment gap is an ongoing process. I challenged myself to confront my own *biases and opinions* and to think openly so I can better understand the *scientific and humanistic* aspects of addictions and their treatments. I was puzzled (and remained throughout my career) to experience the skepticism of the public as well as of the medical community about the nature of addictive disorders and the effectiveness of their treatments despite our society being fully aware of the seriousness of drug and alcohol-related issues such as driving fatalities, overdoses, child abuse and neglect, and overutilization of medical and emergency services, to name just a few.

How did the process of my personal transformation start and of finding a career path develop?

Reflecting on my training in medical school, I remember what fascinated me was listening to the stories of my patients in which their struggles and suffering played out in front of my eyes. What a humbling experience! I knew early on that I wanted to make a difference in patients' lives. This inspired me to embark on a challenging journey to learn more about how to do just that and discover what it means to be a healer. Stephen Levine's [5] statement resonated with me:

> *If there is a single definition of healing, it is to enter with mercy and awareness those pains, mental and physical, from which we have withdrawn in judgment and dismay.*

Living by and practicing these words are naturally complicated and challenging. Genuineness is essential and among the most important attributes of a healer [6]. As medical students, we were taught to "take the history" and "examine the patient" so we can formulate a diagnosis. William Osler once noted: "Listen to the patient: he is telling you the diagnosis." Another approach inextricably associated with listening to the patient emphasizes a paradoxical angle: "taking the patient" (being with the patient and accepting the patient) and "examining the history" (immersing yourself in examining their life with them). This approach transforms the therapeutic encounter into a healing and "growth-fostering" connection [7].

I realized in my first months of training in psychiatry in the early 1990s how important it was to engage *emotionally* with my patients and doing it "now." I was not willing to wait for the distant days of more experience and "qualifications." Indeed, I did not wait. I started the process of learning to listen, expanding my knowledge in basic therapeutic skills, practicing and honing them, and receiving guidance and supervision from my mentors. In fact, my personal transformation started with learning to *just listen*. I remember in my first year of residency training picking up one of my favorite readings: *Talking Sense* by the great medical essayist Richard Asher. He was a physician at the Central Middlesex Hospital during the 1950s and 1960s. Asher described himself as "a physician more at home at the bedside than in the laboratory." He advocated for the importance of "experience and noticing" and asserted that doctors need to think for themselves and trust their own senses and intuition. Clinical observation skills are very important and ever improvable. I have made it my focus to strengthen mine throughout my career. What struck me was his emphasis on the importance of experience—*Experientia docet* ("Experience teaches")—validating the fact that "many things which in theory ought to be highly effective turn out in practice to be completely useless" [8].

My own personal twist on Asher's perspective is that the experience of listening teaches too and teaches well. Clearly, listening and empathy are intertwined; to be able to empathize one must listen genuinely, and to listen genuinely one must approach the other in an empathic stance. I remember as a new trainee in psychotherapy becoming cognizant of the importance of focusing on empathy as a fundamental [9], if not sufficient, "condition" for patient change [10]. Kohut [11] defined empathy as "vicarious introspection," with its overtones of looking inside on behalf of someone else. For him, empathy was itself the method of psychotherapy; for me empathy is a *sine qua non* of any psychotherapeutic approach. The core readings in my initial efforts to become a clinician who might one day become a healer were by Carl Rogers [12, 13]. I was then as I have been ever since "a pupil of Rogers." It has been shown that much of the positive impact of psychotherapeutic approaches comes not specifically from the credentials and expertise of the practitioner, but from what Rogers [12] described as the practitioner's way of being: the practitioner's mindset and corresponding interpersonal stance and interaction. Rogers and his student Charles Truax [14] theoretically defined one such therapist-provided condition—"accurate empathy"—as "the ability of the therapist accurately and sensitively to understand experiences of feelings and *their meanings to the client* during the moment-to-moment encounter of psychotherapy" (p. 104). As Rogers described empathy as a "way of being," idiosyncratic to every psychotherapeutic relationship, he also asserted that *his* way of being empathic was to listen reflectively. I knew early on that I wanted his way of being with patients to be my way. Indeed, Rogers stressed the importance of accordance between the therapist's way of being and his or her beliefs and values. This book is as much about that humanism (that has never been said any better since Rogers!) as it is about blending it with the science of addiction that has become a part of addiction treatment in the intervening decades.

As part of a psychotherapy film series made in the 1960s, Rogers interviewed a patient named Gloria who was so affected by how well she had been heard by Rogers that she stayed in touch with him until the day she died some 25 years later. The powerful impact was related to being heard, once, for 30 min! As a budding clinician, listening reflectively was for me a new skill. All I was familiar with was *attentive/passive listening*. As I recall first learning, all that I needed to do was to simply let the patient talk while I listened and keep the communication limited to occasional empathic sounds. This style could still convey concern, caring, and acceptance. Well, not exactly! Then I discovered *Active Listening*, which was coined by Rogers' student, Thomas Gordon [15]. Active listening means the clinician capturing what the patient means, conveying respect and acceptance, and helping the patient to better understand her own internal processes—thoughts, feelings, associations—and to express them openly in a safe atmosphere.

My experiences of actively listening led me to learn new ways of entering the orbit of the patient's experiences. My early practice of active listening, however, was hugely challenged by a longstanding belief in maintaining an interpersonal distance from the patient and relying more on the cognitive and intellectual aspects than the emotional dynamic of the therapeutic relationship. Throughout medical school training and even in residency training, I was encouraged to learn to stay emotionally detached if I was to provide objective medical care and prevent burnout. Initially, I thought this made sense. I remember being told as a doctor that I can still act effectively, with compassion, but without the risk of emotional overinvolvement with my patients; the operative stance was to "distance yourself from sorrow and maintain affective neutrality." Moreover, my earliest training as a psychiatrist occurred in the context of rigid traditional psychodynamic theories and frameworks, prescribing a neutral and passive response to patients' emotional pain and struggles. It was a well-intentioned approach, but one which left me wanting more meaning. I was searching for more of an intimate, empathic, in a word, a more healing connection with my patients.

My approach totally changed when I realized how it conflicted with my ability to *be with my patients* during moments of genuine empathic connection; moments in which I could evocatively experience the patients' suffering. This powerful process stimulated my scientific curiosity about patients' struggles with substance use problems on the one hand, and my openness to their painful emotional experiences on the other, leading to a shared journey of mutual influence. The poet Audre Lorde described this process in a letter to her therapist when she wrote: "some part of my journey is yours too" [16].

The shared journey and personal transformation started during my first clinical experiences on the psychiatric unit at the VA hospital in my first year of residency training in psychiatry. I volunteered to work with David, a 30-year-old veteran and married man who presented to the emergency room seeking treatment for his alcohol and opioid use disorders. The first moment I met him, I experienced an instant connection with this stranger, who had never engaged in treatment for his substance use. I tried so hard not to be caught up in portraying some image of myself as "the good psychiatrist" or "the healthy expert" and to not come across as thinking of him as "the fragile patient." I wanted to remain authentic and present with him. I was at once so excited to work with David and terrified to embark on an unpredictable journey. I was given full autonomy and responsibility for working with him. So much of my medical school training had focused on learning about diseases and diagnoses with lab values and X-ray readings, objective numbers, and measurable pathology. When I started immersing myself in his world, I had to formulate an entirely new approach and learn what it meant to "connect emotionally" with a person who was suffering and reaching out for help. Medical school had taught me that so much of being a clinician meant mastering objective approaches to patient care. My experience with David clashed with these lessons as I experienced firsthand how the path to healing was through my own subjectivity as it touched with David's. To me, bringing a non-judgmental attitude and awareness of my patient and myself were fundamental to the process of my working with David and of David teaching me how to help him with his own healing.

Early in the moments of our first session, David expressed a powerful desire to change. He shared openly his intention to do it and reclaim his life. *Actively listening* to him, I was so preoccupied with staying "real": genuine, honest, kind, open, and compassionate. My approach was to "just shut up, focus, and listen actively." He was completely engaged despite his physical discomfort with symptoms related to withdrawal from alcohol. I felt deeply privileged to have been "the one" that this man opened up to in his first experience with the healthcare system. I was concerned about what I could do "to hold the relationship" and wondered how he perceived me. We quickly established a working relationship where we trusted each other. Additionally, I started collaborating with his social worker to help him with resources and with obtaining access to VA benefits that he was not aware even existed. Our second day in treatment started out with him perseverating on the detoxification protocol with diazepam for alcohol withdrawal symptoms, requesting a bigger dose, and making threats that he can act like "a fool." I felt intimidated and thought to myself, "he must be going through a horrible experience of withdrawal and we are not doing enough to effectively treat him given his history of drinking more than a gallon of liquor daily." I reassured David that we would do our best to manage his symptoms and explore his inability to cope with physical complaints, negative emotions, and his use of alcohol to self-soothe these emotions. He was an open and willing man as he started incorporating skills for self-management of his anxiety. He was grateful for the work we were doing together.

During our next session, David continued to be focused on his physical symptoms which I felt impeded having a more effective working relationship. I fretted that his focus on his various complaints blocked us from exploring his struggles with alcohol and opioids, which seemed to me to be so clearly linked to traumatic experiences he had in his early life as a child. Our discussion tended to shift towards medication treatments which I believed distracted from delving deeper into his struggles. He shared that his wife had been expecting to visit him later that day and he was excited about it. I proposed to schedule a meeting with all three of us to better understand the impact of his substance use on his life and his relationship with his wife, to advance to a conversation about treatment options following his discharge from the hospital. He reiterated how grateful he was for my investment in his recovery. My sense of hope was renewed that he could cope better with his struggles and engage more in treatment. I was optimistic for him and prepared for what we could discuss in the joint session with his wife.

During the morning report the next day, I was informed of a series of events. First, his wife's visit ended abruptly after he got into an argument with her and attacked her verbally. Then, the staff reported that almost half an hour after the visit, David showed signs of possible drug intoxication. I struggled with anger as I wondered whether our management of his withdrawal from alcohol could have precipitated his behaviors. Moreover, my session with him and his wife ended up being cancelled since he told us she got into a car accident. I felt angry, disappointed, and confused as I felt our connection being destroyed. As David's behaviors on the unit became more concerning, I attempted many times to reengage him and encourage him to disclose what contributed to his intoxication. In response, he became more distant, evasive, and dismissive as he adamantly denied ingesting any substances. While our team judged that it was counter-therapeutic to keep him in treatment since he was not willing to "come clean" about his behaviors, I was puzzled over the decision to discharge him.

As I re-approached him with these concerns, he became angry and stated that he did not feel "safe" to leave because he couldn't trust himself not to hurt his wife. When I asked him to clarify what he meant, he coolly articulated "you'll find out tonight." I was worried that his comment was an implicit threat to his wife's safety. After a contemplative pause, he shared that he was "pushing my buttons," that he never had any intent to hurt her. He said that he was full of rage because she did not understand "his pain." I became more confused and continued to question whether discharging him was the best option. I became aware that his first experience in treatment might affect his perception of the healthcare system. I worried how it could breed resentment and a reluctance to seek treatment in the future when perhaps he was more willing. Soon after, the team decided to proceed with his discharge. David decided he wanted to be "honest with you [me] because you [I] care" and disclosed to me that he indeed took two pills of an opioid that he sneaked into the unit. I was relieved, less bewildered, and encouraged as I saw this encounter as a step towards his reengaging in treatment. It felt so personal to me. I thought this turn by David could potentially change our approach towards his treatment. But it was too late: the unit had a clear zero tolerance policy regarding the use of illicit substances on the unit; the decision to discharge him was non-negotiable.

I felt deeply conflicted about this decision since I thought it was an opportunity. I thought that we should give him another chance to work with us. The staff bluntly countered that he was "not ready" and that he therefore should leave. I was not convinced that he was "unmotivated" to change! Regardless of my perspective, the team's decision to discharge him was firm. After his departure, I wondered "what there must be" in his inner world that he was not able to disclose. My experience of working with him put me back in touch with my own feelings: starting off being hopeful and excited about making a difference in someone's life who after so long finally took the first steps to seek help, and ending up feeling upset, terrified, confused, disappointed, and insecure. Sorting through this experience and my own psychic turmoil was a transformative experience for me! Later, I decided to reread some sections in the book *The Doctor, His Patient and the Illness* [17] written by the psychoanalyst Michael Balint who mentioned that the most important therapy at the doctor's disposal was the doctor himself. What matters is the relationship with the patient and the dynamics of this relationship. Balint and Balint [18] noted:

> *Knowledge can be learned from books and lectures; skill must be acquired by doing the thing, and its price in psychotherapy must always be a limited though considerable change of one's own personality. Without this, psychotherapy, so-called, is a well-intentioned, amateurish exercise; it is this change of personality that raises it to a professional level.*

Through this early though deeply formative experience with David, I could see how working to help a patient change meant being open to allowing the experience to change me in a personal way, too. I believe that the turmoil and bewilderment that I endured on a personal level during this work with David was crucial to understanding in a deeper and a more empathic way David's struggles on the unit. I believe that those moments during which I thought David would turn around and reengage were no less possible because of the way I was learning to work through my own internal conflicts in trying to be a empathic healer. I did not know at that time how my experience of my own fumbling and moments of doubt would become so critical to a journey towards transformation, including the acquisition of the skills so integral to healing. It was only through more experiences like this and my own reflections on their meanings that I have been able to see (and feel!) the experiential ingredients of learning to heal. It is *this stuff* that I have learned on this personal and sometimes painful journey that is *the stuff* of this book.

Speaking of which: I must continue to share with you what I call the *epiphanies* of my own journey during my early career. I have never seen greater courage, hope, and resilience than when Shannon began sharing with me her world that is filled with pain, sorrow, and suffering. One night previously she had walked into the emergency room alone requesting admission to the psychiatric unit and told the staff that her depression and heroin use were getting so bad that she felt she would kill herself by overdosing if she didn't get help. There she was, sitting in the treatment room, her very first inpatient experience, in front of me, who followed her every word. I wanted to convey to her that "we are in this together," so I could listen actively, truly be with her, join her in her world, and understand her as a person, and not just an "utterer of symptoms." I tried to envision what I would feel like at that moment if I were her: what would I do if I was asked to explore feelings I'd spent the better part of my life trying to get away from? How could I trust if this stranger is trying to understand me or judge me? I was terrified. I realized that any disclosure by her must evoke a response from me, but I was not sure I knew how to be open to what she had to share. It struck me: how could I ask her to share openly if I was not willing to be open and affected in as deep a way as I wanted her to be in sharing with me? How could I be at ease with her if I am not at ease with myself? I began to see that there had to be more symmetry in our relatedness if her sharing was to be easier, deeper, and more meaningful. I felt as vulnerable as I searched trepidatiously within myself for the words that could convey my openness and be as inviting and safe for her as possible: "Help me understand what you've been going through? What made you decide to seek help?" Her answer startled me with its clarity and poignancy: "Since my father died, I feel like I've been going crazy." She shared what she'd been going through during the prior weeks, and at the same time I could see her holding back. She wasn't used to letting her emotions into the light. They were building up and choking her. But she felt like she might be "crazy," and if I were her I would have felt very vulnerable sharing that. I said, "These are painful experiences you're sharing, and when we share our fears like you're doing it can leave us feeling vulnerable. I appreciate how hard you're trying to be open with me even though it's difficult. We are here to work together through this process." Her eye contact dramatically improved after this statement. With each reflective listening statement and each validation of her struggles, she felt more understood, and she trusted she could let me into her world and still be safe; I appreciated how a small, meaningful statement could make an enormous impact on our relationship. I saw our conversations as a series of small yet significant successes; they were steps forward in forging an emotional connection. I encouraged her to *share anything*; I worked hard *to hear anything*. I had never appreciated to what extent my presence and *openness* with her could shape the course of her initial treatment experience, although I had been aware for quite some time of what the research tells us: a positive initial experience with the mental healthcare system predicts greater chance of long-term engagement and retention in services; a negative one can be disastrous. I considered how my own being, attitude, tone of voice, and words could influence these crucial initial moments of engagement. I scrutinized every listening statement, every question, and "the putting of every question," all of which significantly positively influenced the responses I sought to gather from Shannon and other patients. My goal of improving these points of contact became an effort to improve my construction of each sentence and response to be more inviting, more person-centered, and more collaborative. Focusing on achieving small successes and learning from the challenges, we spent more time in individual work. I believe we were affecting each other and changing each other by the process of mutual influence: she shifted from relating facts and I shifted from collecting data about how much she was using—snorting 30 bags of heroin, drinking a pint of alcohol daily—to opening up about what she believed using the drugs really did for her. Namely, she shared that she used these substances to numb the intolerable grief and self-hate she had been experiencing ever since her father died unexpectedly a year ago. It was only then that I experienced a different dimension of knowing her as a person versus knowing about her. Her feelings were very intense. I found that it took a lot of effort for me to sit with her and listen without trying to come up with solutions. She sobbed most of the time we were talking. She blamed herself for her father's death (in fact due to severe heart disease) as she had been his primary caretaker until a few months before his death. He had decided to move out at that point, and she subsequently blamed herself for allowing him to live on his own. She was there almost daily for the first month after he moved out, yet she still blamed herself for not checking in on him enough. When he got sick and required admission to the hospital, Shannon gathered up some of his clothes from his apartment to bring to him. Sadly, she arrived only to see him take his last breaths before dying. She was struggling with deep self-blame. She felt that if she had gotten there sooner she could have done something. She described to me her intrusive thoughts of her father throughout the day which were nothing more to her than reminders of how she "caused" his death. Every time she felt like she could feel some purpose or had some momentary hope, thoughts of her father and images of his death would pop into her head; she ruminated on how she failed him, felt overwhelming guilt and worthlessness, and fell into a depressive abyss. She read his obituary throughout each day and had it on the fridge because she felt it meant he was still there with her.

Her depression and thoughts to kill herself began only after his death. She had never snorted heroin until a week after he died and she hadn't stopped since. The intensity of her grief was unchanged from the moment he died, and she felt she was "crazy" to still be feeling the pain that intensely. "What's wrong with me?" she wondered. She finally expressed why she had not sought treatment until she was sure she would kill herself if she didn't: she feared being labeled as "crazy" for how she mentally fell apart after her father's death and had been unable to "get over it."

For many patients, financial, geographic, and awareness barriers impede engagement in services. Alternatively, working with Shannon made me realize how destructive the barrier of stigma can be. I spent considerable time with her normalizing her feelings: the pain of the loss does not go away, yet, typically, people can integrate it into their lives in a way that makes sense to them and allows them to continue with their efforts to attain their daily and long-term goals. However, Shannon never had the chance to work through her grief to be able to integrate it, as she had numbed it with drugs right after her father died. This perspective resonated with her: she hadn't had a chance to grieve properly. Why had she been so desperate to numb the grief? Why was she only able to connect with the pain but not to the love that she shared with her father? I didn't fully understand these questions at that point, and we hadn't had enough small successes to allow her to feel safe enough to disclose the reasons that kept her from taking the next steps.

However, with each further small gain in working together, Shannon shared more about her life. The truth was she had been struggling long before her father's death. Her depression began in childhood. She had been using drugs since she was 15, starting with abusing prescription painkillers, alcohol, and marijuana. Both her parents were addicted to heroin when she was young. I could see how my empathic listening corrected for the lack of or disrupted "mirroring" which she received from her parents. She had never been taught to use or observe others using skills for managing emotions without substances. Then she revealed what no one else outside of her family knew: her father had been physically and verbally abusive to her throughout her childhood. Only later in her life did he come to understand his own feelings and actions, and mend their relationship. She was unable to separate her anger at losing him from her anger over the abuse.

I struggled for a way to reframe the loss for her and was not confident in exploring strategies to do so. I expressed these concerns to my mentor, who guided me through the process. With his help, I was ultimately able to reframe her father's moving out of her apartment as his way of growing up as a man and getting out on his own. This separation was something her father needed to do for himself. Shannon was more comfortable with this conceptualization of the events leading up to his death; she came to accept that her father was more at peace when he died and that she was not responsible for his death. Because of her positive experiences with us on the unit, Shannon decided she wanted to continue in specialized grief counseling after discharge. She had already begun to reconnect with positive memories of her father and wanted to continue this work. After 7 days in inpatient treatment, she transitioned to a partial outpatient program, decided to engage in grief therapy, was taking an antidepressant regularly, knew exactly which Narcotics Anonymous (NA) meetings she would be attending every day, and was working on the steps with her sponsor.

I learned a great deal from my work with Shannon that I would continue to use to transform my future encounters with patients. I gained an appreciation of how the small successes in communication and listening actively shape the patient-doctor relationship (how I had to be personally present to influence the treatment outcomes), overcome the power of stigma which stymies people in need from reaching out and foster the healing process. When I used to think about what kind of treatment it would take to make a difference in a person's life, I pictured rehabs, mutual support groups, psychotropic medications, and detoxification protocols. Perhaps the most impactful thing that Shannon taught me was that it is the connection that truly matters most, and that connection depends in part on my own openness to the patient, to myself, and to being changed by the process itself. In our final session, she told me that *our relationship* made her feel safe to unload her grief, to share the trauma that she had disclosed with no one, and that now she felt like she can trust others to help her, and that is what gave her hope. She thanked me for sitting with her all those hours while she cried for not running away from her tears and her suffering: "Thank you for helping me to understand myself and for the work we did together." Her courage and resilience showed me I had the courage to be more open and at ease with myself.

Erikson [19] noted that "we cannot lift a case history out of history," by which he meant: (1) You cannot ignore the significance of the exact details and facts of the patient's history: what the patient shares in his or her own words is inextricably linked to factors of place and time and is so much more important than just the expression of almost monosyllabic notes such as depressed, anxious, etc.; and (2) It is the sense of history which acts as a background to the patient's clinical history.

Working with Shannon taught me that the experience of therapeutic listening is transformative and filled with intense astonishment and unpredictability. To me, listening empathically feels spiritual. Buber [20] emphasized that the essence of spirituality consisted of a "meeting" between the "I" of one with the "Thou" of another, and empathy makes it happen. To genuinely be present and listening to Shannon, to create a quiet therapeutic space and to minimize distractions, to enter her complex internal experiences, and hear her share her struggles and conflicts as well as her potential: all of these elements made for a powerful process that has many similarities with meditation. It was an ultimate state of being present and open to Shannon's experience. It is so difficult to put this into words. It is for me as close as I have come to a divine encounter.

I am sharing the next clinical piece because it made me learn about the challenges of the uncertainty of clinical judgment. In fact, I expected more certainty of myself. I also wished to be more knowledgeable and secure. This is not realistic. It also made me realize that, however clear and simple the patients' psychological conflicts may appear to be, most of the time there is an underlying deeper complexity to their struggles that may remain difficult to uncover. Experiencing the patients' dilemmas does not mean that one should also look for a way to fix their problems. The lesson to learn was to strive to become a *better* physician with time and more experience. While I was not attempting psychoanalysis, I recalled the work of Bion [21] who had said that "the psychoanalyst needs to be able to question himself as often as and as long as he is unsatisfied, but should not spend too much looking for the answers in books. The time we have is limited: we must read people."

Sean was another person, a "book" from whom I would learn so much about addiction, its treatment, and what sort of psychiatrist I wanted to become. He was admitted on a Wednesday on the dual diagnosis unit for suicidal ideation in the setting of heavy multi-substance drug use. When he arrived, he said that he didn't want to go on living the way that he had been: self-medicating depression, grief, and anger, for half of his life with alcohol and heroin. He had made several attempts at recovery in the past and had been intermittently successful at maintaining sobriety. He talked about periods of months and even longer when he had not used any drugs. During some of these periods, he said he chaired NA meetings and even sponsored others struggling with addiction. At the same time, he found himself always drawn back to using, most recently after he had back surgery and was prescribed opioid painkillers. From his experience in NA, he had developed a sense of what people needed to do to be successful in their recovery; this time, he said, he knew he would need to go to an inpatient residential program, would need to do a "90 in 90" (90 meetings in 90 days) through NA, and would need to address the underlying emotional struggles that kept him stuck in the cycles of addiction that he had never truly worked on. I was optimistic and hopeful from the start that, working together, Sean and I might be able to get to the bottom of his struggles related to his addiction.

Through listening actively, I learned more about where Sean was coming from as a person. His father had left his family and then died when he was a child. He had been physically abused by a stepfather when he was a teenager, was subsequently kicked out of his house for acting out, and sent to a forensic housing program. He was able to complete culinary school and worked as a chef in several restaurants. He had been in and out of halfway and three-quarter houses, and had consequently moved up and down the East Coast. He had once been engaged, but his fiancée had died unexpectedly in a boating accident. He had never addressed his grief surrounding this loss, instead turning to more intense drug use. He had stolen from and had hurt his family to support his drug use and, at times, simply to be "vindictive." He had been in prison, as he had gotten into the habit of borrowing people's cars and not returning them. At the time he entered treatment he was also homeless. He was struggling more with anger, scared by the fact that he "enjoyed" beating up an acquaintance for making passes at an underage girl. Although he reported his mother had always been supportive of him, the fact that he was so adamant that she be called by our staff to be told that he was in recovery spoke to the fact that he was beginning to question this.

Despite the circumstances of our lives being very different, I felt connected to Sean. He was affable and had a good sense of humor. His life had been extremely difficult, but he was well traveled and had many fascinating life stories and experiences. For the first couple of days of his experience in treatment, Sean was well engaged in working together and in the therapeutic activities on the unit. He and I discussed openly and in depth his struggles and he identified areas which he wanted to work on or explore. He specifically requested the opportunity to share about his fiancée's death in our Friday individual session, during which he was grateful to spend more than an hour with me. I felt I was getting to know him and more about him, and I was at this point highly invested in his work on recovery.

As his experience in treatment went on over the course of the following week, though, he became less engaged and more detached from me. He began to fraternize heavily with the some of the female patients on the unit who were in his age range, and, at the same time due to poor sleep, he no longer had the energy to have productive afternoon treatment sessions or even focus during shorter ones. He skipped group activities "to catch up on sleep." His poor sleep and withdrawal symptoms became his focus and he declined another opportunity to talk about grief on Friday, as he felt like he would "regress" emotionally and was already too uncomfortable physically. "I'm having an off day," he explained. I was most surprised when, on Monday morning, he requested to be discharged and stated that he would go to outpatient treatment. He felt he had accomplished everything he could in treatment at this point, he explained, and he said he was ready to go on to the next step. I was confused. Hadn't he wanted to go to an inpatient residential program? Hadn't he wanted to work on his emotional struggles and coping? What did he feel he accomplished after the first couple of days? Where was he going to find someone who would spend a lot of time working with him? That afternoon, Sean admitted to me that he was planning to leave and start using again. Yet, he also was having second thoughts, realizing that leaving treatment now could be another time of "running away" from his problems. He said his withdrawal symptoms were just so difficult to tolerate. I expressed that I would see what we could do to manage his withdrawal symptoms. "I really wanted to stay in treatment," he said in a way that did not feel so authentic to me. He talked briefly about his fiancée's death, but then he said he was getting too physically uncomfortable which ended our session. The next day, after agreeing for several minutes that his intention was to continue working on his recovery and pursue a residential program, even if it was to be uncomfortable, Sean sat dejected over the news that his detoxification medications were to be discontinued since he completed the taper. In response, he said, he would prefer to leave.

What happened? I had the opportunity to work with a patient who presented as highly motivated, had a great amount of insight into why he was struggling, had a clear plan about what his recovery plan was after discharge, and had been willing to work with me. Yet the result was that he left before addressing the problems that he himself had identified; he made the very decision that he had once identified to me as running away from his problems.

I doubted myself: what was wrong about my approach? Was I not good enough somehow? Did I miss something all along? What could I have done differently such that he would have stayed in treatment and worked on recovery? If treating addiction is a matter of life and death, did I cost this man his life? Somehow I felt responsible for his decisions, but even this feeling did not seem quite right to me. Many questions went through my mind: I've spent a lot of time thinking about this patient, and I work through some of these questions in a kind of psychiatric "Morbidity and Mortality conference." What I do know for sure is that I wanted to help him, that I was available to work with him, and that I was invested in his success and well-being. I know that he at least mentioned that working with me was one of the most helpful aspects of his treatment experience. I know he was grateful for the work we did together. At the same time, I also know that there are people more experienced with addiction treatment than I am. And I'm still frustrated with this outcome, given where he started. I wish I had a second chance, or maybe that he had a second chance in treatment with someone else. In working through this experience with Sean, I came to see that I was responsible for my role in the treatment of Sean and his ailments; I was not responsible for what Sean chose to do about the treatment. This realization clarified for me what I had to focus on being most helpful to the people I was discovering I wanted to spend my career helping. To be most helpful to them in reclaiming their own lives, I had to be invested in the process of treatment and healing itself. I could only hold myself responsible for a patient's decision about treatment when I was falling short of being the best healer that I could be.

After this experience with Sean, the biggest question became "where do I go from here?" How invested do I allow myself to "be with patients?" How do I change and grow from this experience? How can I make decisions in the presence of uncertainty and incomplete knowledge? The only way that I saw to erase the sense of self-doubt that I've experienced from working with this patient was to continue my clinical practice relying on strengthening my listening skills, learning from patients, and growing with experience. Not being invested in a patients' well-being is clearly never an option. Struggling emotionally with my patients would enrich my own experience in providing care and help me to find my own inner spirit. Should my feelings be hurt and my clinical judgment be questioned when a patient decides to do something with which I do not agree? That isn't a particularly healthy or sustainable attitude either. I needed to work on finding balance between wanting patients to do well and recognizing that I cannot control their decisions. Respecting patient autonomy was a huge lesson for me. I also had to accept that, just maybe, I would not always know what is "best" for them.

Sean was, most likely, making the decision to return to a way of life that he had known for the entirety of his adulthood. The things that he was still trying to cope with were, no doubt, painful for him to think about, re-experience, and work through. I cannot begin to imagine the many losses and traumas that he had to endure. He found out that people were less willing to help him than they had been in the past; when he did contact his mother, she said she did not want to be in touch with him until he had achieved at least 12 months in recovery. Maybe, from his perspective, this experience in treatment allowed him to spend some time talking about struggles that were bothering him with someone that "was present and just listened" and cared about him. Maybe identifying and starting to face his emotional struggles and his addiction this time would help him to start opening up about them and dealing with them during his next treatment experience. As he articulated, his recovery was entirely up to him at this point.

Next, I am sharing a humbling clinical experience I had with Daniel. I was able to be open to the "unknown" in him and about him and willing to find out. Instead of using short cuts, we jointly discovered what was needed to make working together therapeutic. Bion [21] noted that when a therapist learns to follow the patient's cues and listens to the resulting dialogue between the two viewpoints of "binocular vision" of knowing and not knowing, the result is a better understanding of the patient and his or her struggles.

Before even coming up to the dual diagnosis unit, Daniel's reputation preceded him. One of the first words I heard in passing used to describe him was that he was a "psychopath," and none of the staff wanted him on our unit. He had been brought in by the police for an involuntary commitment for brandishing firearms and repeatedly threatening to kill people, and he had even made threats to kill staff in the emergency room. I reviewed his records to get a better idea of "the person" behind these behaviors. In my review, I found plenty of judgmental interpretations about his past and present legal issues and very few statements from, or discussions with, the patient himself. He was labeled as "noncompliant" with medications and treatments and "difficult" because he didn't listen or care. It was hard not to jump to conclusions, and I formed a pretty fixed conceptualization about him before we had ever met. I admit that I, too, thought of him as a "monster" and had no idea how to even prepare myself. To say I was surprised when I met Daniel would be an understatement.

Daniel was a gray-haired man in his late fifties, limping with the help of a walker. He was cordial and pleasant with me, practically the opposite of what I had expected. He didn't look like a "monster" nor act like one in any way. I could tell right away that I had made a serious mistake in being so stigmatizing and judgmental. I felt guilty, ashamed, and at the same time humbled by my mistake. I realized that I did not know anything at all about this man, his life, or the struggles that he was going through. I had been thinking so much about how I would deal with a potentially "aggressive patient" or how I would have a working relationship with a patient labeled with an antisocial personality disorder that I completely forgot to think about getting to know who *he* is, what *he* had been going through to end up on the unit, or what *he* wanted to change. Everything I had been preparing in my head was suddenly worthless and my sense of self fell down several notches as I began to feel like I might not be good at working therapeutically with patients. Daniel, however, was willing to talk with me, and since I no longer had an agenda, I could actively listen to him and try to get to know him. It was hard to clear the things I had heard from my head and not think of him in terms of the diagnoses in his old records. At the same time, all I had to do was listen to what he was sharing and where he was coming from. When he asked about his involuntary commitment, I simply admitted that I had heard a lot of things about him from others. It was remarkable to see how well he responded when I honestly told him that, despite what I had heard about him, I did not know him at all, and I hoped we could work together. As it turned out, he could explain his behaviors very coherently and offered a reasonable perspective without trying to make excuses. He took responsibility and regretted his actions that had resulted in the involuntary commitment, and at the same time his situation was very clearly a product of an environment most people do not understand. He did not want to shoot anyone or even hurt anyone; he was just terrified and concerned about his safety with the violence around him all his life. In the past year, he was stabbed five times in his own home so severely that he needed to be hospitalized. Additionally, his struggles with alcohol use resulted in episodes where he blacked out and lost control of his temper. He was just as afraid of these incidents as other people had been because he knew himself to be a nonviolent person who did not own guns nor want to shoot anyone. He was extremely hard on himself and very demoralized by his inability to control his drinking and ultimately by his inability to control his behaviors. He openly identified some issues he wanted to work on including coping with his anger, managing his depression, and controlling his drinking. He was grateful to be getting the treatment he knew he needed and wanted because he had been unable to seek it out on his own. It was clear to me that Daniel had not been given the chance to share what mattered to him and find out what he wanted to work on. He was genuinely surprised that I respected him as "a person." Instead of setting him on the defensive, I met him where he was, and he then brought out his own willingness to change. He gave me the opportunity to learn a lot more about his values and his reasons for wanting to change. For a patient who was supposedly "noncompliant" and "difficult," he was well engaged in treatment. Working with Daniel taught me a lot about interacting not with patients but with people in general. I thought I would not be able to engage him because of my own preconceptions, and, if I had maintained that attitude, I truly never would have been able to work with him. Furthermore, it would not have been his issue; it would have been mine. Daniel wanted to work with me even though we were separated by a lifetime of unique and different experiences, and he taught me that all I needed to do was to accept him for who he was and be present with him. This clinical experience made me realize that it is inevitable to make mistakes. Nevertheless, in this stumbling it was Daniel who made me discover what I then stumbled upon, by allowing me to work with him.

A recurrent theme of this book is learning from my own mistakes, how to avoid them as best I can, how to become better aware of those times when I am judgmental or form an opinion of somebody without knowing anything about them. Such experiences have and continue to be profoundly mutually therapeutic and healing for my patients and myself.

Many more lessons have emerged from my early experiences working with patients with addictions. Practicing honesty was fundamentally at the core of my interactions with them. Before engaging in therapeutic conversations, I always assess my thoughts and impulses, making sure I filter how I communicate the truth tactfully, honestly, and respectfully without jeopardizing my relationship with patients. To me, respect means that I experience other people as they truly are, listening to their struggles, and genuinely attempting to understand their perspectives without criticizing, judging, or putting them down. Above all, these formative experiences lead me to make a commitment to be honest with myself and reflect on my own insecurities and self-doubt instead of focusing on other people's flaws and vulnerabilities, both in my work and my personal life. Throughout the journey of developing my empathic skills, I discovered that empathy and humility are intimately connected. I worked hard to control being self-critical and remind myself that I have so many opportunities to learn, experience, and make mistakes. I entered every therapeutic encounter with an open mind that gave me the chance to set aside my own biases and not allow them to obstruct my ability to be empathic. This open mind is well articulated by the beginner's mind that Zen practitioners defined as a mind innocent of preconceptions, expectations, judgments, and prejudices: *"in the beginner's mind there are many possibilities, but in the expert's there are few"* [22]. During my training, in addition to keeping up with the open mindedness that I discussed above, I have pursued a cultivation of the Zen spirit in my clinical practice and life through practicing meditation and mindfulness. I will share its impact on my career in Chap. 2.

References

1. Walant KB. Creating the capacity for attachment: treating addictions and the alienated self. Northwale, NJ: Jason Aronson Inc.; 1995.
2. Miller WR, Rollnick S. Motivational interviewing: preparing people to change addictive behavior. New York: Guilford Press; 1991.
3. Wilson B. Alcoholics anonymous: the story of how more than one hundred men have recovered from alcoholism. 2nd ed: The Anonymous Press; 1955.
4. Marlatt GA, Gordon JR. Relapse prevention: maintenance strategies in the treatment of addictive disorders. New York: Guilford Publication; 1985.
5. Levine S. A year to live: how to live this year as if it were your last. New York: Bell Tower; 1998.
6. Truax C, Carkhuff R. Towards effective counseling and psychotherapy: training and practice. New York: Aldine Publications; 1967.
7. Miller JB, Stiver IP. The healing connection: how women form relationships in therapy and life. Boston: Beacon Press; 1997.
8. Asher R. Apriority: thoughts on treatment. Lancet. 1961;2(7217):1403–4.
9. Kohut H. The analysis of the self. New York: International Universities Press; 1989.
10. Rogers CR. The necessary and sufficient conditions of therapeutic personality change. J Consult Psychol. 1957;21(2):95–103.
11. Kohut H. Introspection, empathy, and psychoanalysis: an examination of the relation between mode of observation and theory. J Am Psychoanal Assoc. 1957;7:459–83.
12. Rogers CR. Client-centered therapy. Washington, DC: American Psychological Association; 1966.

References

13. Rogers CR. A way of being. Boston: Houghton Mifflin; 1995.
14. Rogers CR, Truax CB. The therapeutic conditions antecedent to change: a theoretical view. In: Rogers CR, Gendlin ET, Kiesler DJ, Truax CB, editors. The therapeutic relationship and its impact: a study of psychotherapy with schizophrenics. Madison: University of Wisconsin Press; 1967.
15. Gordon T. Parent effectiveness training: the proven program for raising responsible children. New York: Three Rivers Press; 1970.
16. Lorde A. Sister outsider. Freedom, CA: The Crossing Press; 1984.
17. Balint M. The doctor, his patient and the illness. London: Pitman Medical; 1963.
18. Balint M, Balint E. Psychotherapeutic techniques in medicine. Abingdon, UK: Routledge; 2002.
19. Erikson EH. Young man Luther. London: Faber and Faber; 1950.
20. Buber M. Existential guilt. In: Smith RW, editor. Smith, guilt, man, and society. New York: Anchor Books; 1971.
21. Bion WR. Brasilia clinical seminars. In: Bion F, editor. Clinical seminars and four papers. Abingdon, UK: Fleetwood Press; 1987.
22. Suzuki S. Zen mind, beginner's mind. New York: Weatherhill; 1980.

Chapter 2
Cultivating Empathy and Emotional Openness in Practice

> *"May we open to deeper understanding*
> *And a genuine love and caring*
> *For the multitude of faces*
> *Who are none other than ourself."*
>
> —Wendy Egyoku Nakao

Being empathic is itself considered an evidence-based practice [1]. The American Psychological Association Task Force on Evidence-based Therapy Relationships [2] has designated empathy as an evidence-based element of the therapeutic relationship and has recommended that training programs incorporate curricula focusing on the relationship elements of clinical practice.

Describing my own experience cultivating empathy skills in my clinical career helps me reflect on how I have evolved and matured in my capacity and identity as a healer. My training in motivational interviewing (MI) coincided with my exposure to learning and practicing Zen Buddhism. At the core of each of these practices for me was working to change my entire mental foundation for better listening. The process started with focusing on my *self-listening* skills and paying so much attention to my inaccuracies and negative perceptions and distortions about people's perspectives, especially those of my patients. Learning to build my therapeutic language and how I modulate my tone of voice, choose my words, and articulate them into sentences that truly represent what I mean to say, were fundamental to avoiding destructive communication behaviors in clinical encounters. The first step in building myself into a more empathic listener entailed listening to my own inner thoughts and verbal communications while asking what needed to change within so that my mind could become more open to experiencing the other. During these efforts, I experienced more consciously my tendency to become overwhelmed and angry with my patients when they did not engage according to my expectations. In these inner reflections on my own mental processes and verbal utterances, I saw that the source of my frustrations was not within an errant patient but within myself. I realized that these discordant experiences with the other happened because of my failure to listen *mindfully*. Initially in my training I thought of myself as a "good listener," but later I discovered just how deeply I was lacking in this most crucial of therapeutic skills. It was so difficult to be disabused of my pretensions to therapeutic proficiency as I realized that listening with *accurate empathy* is a different skill that requires hard work and practice to learn. To me, listening with accurate empathy looks like mindful listening, which is a mindset involving becoming aware of the barriers one created between him or herself and the patient. Accurate empathy might be said to go one step further: it is listening with a focus and a desire to deeply understand another's perspective.

Most of my ideas and experiences in this chapter have evolved from a mélange of my training in motivational interviewing, studying, and practicing Zen Buddhism. The Zen approach of Buddhism is not intended to conflict with any religious denomination. This mindfulness approach is more of a philosophy about life or science than a religion. In some ways, the Zen approach to meditation and mindfulness could be viewed as techniques for a more mindful practice of another spiritual tradition. The teachings are neither mystical nor articles of faith nor intellectual exercise. In fact, they can be viewed as a guide to how to deal with the behavior of the mind.

To me, learning and practicing these teachings helped me focus better, become more compassionate, and keep myself grounded in my work with patients with addictions. Early in its development, MI was defined as an egalitarian, empathetic "way of being." It was conceptualized as a communication style that uses specific skills and strategies such as reflective listening and shared decision-making in the collaborative engagement with a patient. "To heal requires a relationship marked by equality," said Dr. Lown in his book *The Lost Art of Healing* [3], reflecting the importance of an egalitarian approach in clinical encounters. Learning and practicing MI changed my "robotic" approach to patient care, dissolved my old habits (such as prejudice, arrogance, selfishness) that were destructive to the therapeutic work, and made me humbler, more selfless, and more open-minded. Demanding that I cultivate the spirit within myself transformed my mental focus so that I could better listen to the patients. It demanded that I not tolerate coasting in the clinical ruts that forestall the more intimate connection with the patient struggling with the addiction that is so requisite to the healing process. So, a Zen practice became for me a process of undoing the mechanistic behaviors that kept me distant and disengaged. It taught me to better focus, concentrate, and listen effectively. MI and Zen practices have totally transformed my experiences of empathic reflective listening into opportunities for growth, creativity, and a fulfillment I once would have thought I could never know. Listening with accurate empathy has to come from the heart, body, and mind. When these parts of oneself change in deeper ways, they allow for a unique way of relating to patients.

The best way of exercising and building my mindful listening skills has been in my clinical encounters. The Zen philosophy [4] to listening offers us an initial insight or awakening into our true nature, or *kensho*, which also means *comprehension*. The aim of kensho is to liberate us from the confinement of self-interest that disconnects us from the minds of others. The origins of Zen Buddhism go back 2500 years to India when Gautama Siddhartha, a humble prince, abandoned his life to explore the nature of existence. He experienced the suffering of poor people affected by old age and famine. After meditating for many years, he became *enlightened* and became known as the *Buddha* or the Awakened One. It is important to mention that there are several schools of Buddhism (e.g., Tibetan, Pure, Zen, etc.). After the death of Gautama Buddha, the Mahayana tradition spread to Japan where it became Zen.

The mindfulness teachings of Thich Nhat Hanh's Zen Buddhist philosophy resonated totally with me throughout my training in MI. I have incorporated them into my work with patients in whose presence I struggled deeply, learning tremendously from my mistakes and from the patients' guidance throughout the process. Some of these mindfulness principles include:

- Buddhist teachings as a guiding means to help us learn to look deeply and develop our understanding and compassion;
- Learning and practicing non-attachment from views in order to be open to others' insight and experiences;
- Respecting the rights of others to be different and to choose to believe and how to decide;
- Commitment to finding ways to be with those who suffer so we can understand their situation deeply and help them transform their suffering into compassion, peace, and joy;
- Learning to listen deeply without judging or reacting and refraining from uttering words that can create discord;
- Making every effort to keep communications open and to reconcile and resolve all conflicts, however small [5].

The therapeutic style of MI is clearly different from some stereotypic approaches of practitioners from a different time who worked with patients with addiction using confrontational and "attacking" styles of therapy. The therapeutic style of MI is defined by the spirit of partnership that conveys respect and empathic identification with the patient, acknowledging the patient's personal responsibility and autonomy. Specific therapeutic techniques—such as reflective listening with accurate empathy—as I see it are grounded in mindful listening and facilitate the process of change determined by values, choices, and decisions. To me, the resonances of the motivational interviewing spirit and Zen approaches are clear: MI in action is Zen in action and Zen in action is MI in action. Let me be clear: I profess to be neither an *expert* in Eastern philosophy nor even in MI! However, I have studied, learned, practiced, and applied the MI and Zen approaches in my clinical work. I have used them to adapt to and influence the functioning of healthcare systems that can be prone to contributing to the very suffering of people and families with addictions that they seek to treat. Additionally, the Zen and MI approaches have become a way of living that enabled me to work through my own inner struggles that have kept me from being fulfilled in my own life and relationships and which had exposed my vulnerable self-absorbed side. These approaches to my own life and practice pushed me to better myself and choose a more simple and balanced pathway.

The following patient's story reflects a blending of my MI and Zen skills in action. My experience working with Donald taught me the true meaning of empathic listening.

First, I read the psychiatric evaluation from the emergency room about my patient, Donald, and found myself walking hesitantly to his room, expecting to find an "antisocial monster." Like so many of the other catastrophic stories garnered from my patients who struggle with co-occurring psychiatric and substance use disorders, Donald's history of severe alcohol use disorder was laden with many of the common tragic sequelae. His wife and son had grown tired of peeling him up off the floor day after day and night after night; this past summer they were fed up and finally gave up, kicking him and his bottles out of their home. He suffered a life-threatening gastro-intestinal bleed, finally lost the job he had faithfully worked at for 30 years, and found himself alone and homeless, contemplating the value of his life as he peered over the railing of one of the bridges in the city. Instead of jumping, something "clicked" and he decided to get help. For the first time in his life, *he* decided he could not live like this anymore. He called his sister and arrived at the hospital with nothing but a duffle bag and the determination to begin his recovery.

The "sober" Donald I found was nothing like the person depicted in the note I had read. On the contrary, he was gentle, courteous, and soft-spoken. He was supportive and helpful to his peers on the unit. I realized at that moment that I needed to immediately address my judgmental attitude, prejudices, and preconceived notions about him and his value system. Zen masters refer to these barriers as unwholesome mental formations, mental obscurations, and ignorance [6]. So, I started to open and unclutter my mind and listen to him. He disclosed to me some of the most intimate aspects of his life. He described himself as a "Momma's boy." Donald always had a very close relationship with his mother, who at that point was living into her 90s. He sought comfort and approval from her while growing up because his father could never be bothered with him. Despite his greatest efforts to be the star of the baseball team or help by doing extra chores around the house, he never received praise or acceptance let alone acknowledgment and affirmation from his father. At an early age, his father abandoned the family and Donald, the oldest son of five children. Donald then took it upon himself to provide for his siblings and look after his devastated mother. He worked throughout high school to supplement their meager welfare checks which could barely support their household. Donald shared that he did not feel ready to assume these family responsibilities; he believed he never had role modeling from his father to learn how to be the man of the house. Despite his self-doubt, Donald did his best to provide for the family. Even after his siblings married and moved on with their lives, he continued to care for his "depressed and drunken" mother, as he described her. His resentment at his past circumstances and losses was palpable and understandable.

Donald shared with me his life struggles and identified my presence with him in the sessions as "humbling and healing." Donald's father died without Donald ever truly understanding why his father did not accept him as a child. He learned from this emptiness in his life the importance of being a good father for his own son, but he was never able to shed his beliefs in inadequacy, guilt, and loneliness that he carried within him from the loss of his own father. Throughout his upbringing, Donald never shared with others what he bore deep inside. He had to be strong for his mother and younger siblings, which meant denying himself that relief and suppressing his own deep emotions of loss and pain. Talking with his family about their struggles and the things he did not understand could only add to the pain. He described himself as a "bottler." I took that to mean that he bottled up his own pain. In fact, he meant that he relied on the bottle (alcohol) to help him soothe himself by numbing the pain and depression that hurt so deeply.

Donald recognized that his alcohol use and depression only worsened one another. He soon found himself in a vicious, downward spiral: he felt guilty about his drinking and drank more to avoid the ugliness he saw within himself. Too embarrassed to be around his family, he isolated himself to his room where he became even more depressed and lonely. The only solution he could find was to drink more to try to fill the emptiness that would not go away. Over the years, his siblings urged him to stop drinking and seek help, but he was too "hard-headed" and stubborn to listen. He was afraid to accept the gravity of his illness and acknowledge its ill effects on his family and, most importantly on himself. Through the work *we* were doing, Donald recognized that to recover he needed to accept the caring of other people who wanted him in their lives. He saw that he needed to accept the connections from those who wanted to help him face his illness, share his feelings and struggles with others, and take each step one at a time.

Donald challenged himself through the recovery process. He worked through his past experiences, learned about himself in deep emotional ways, and gazed forward towards what he needed to do during his rehabilitation. As the end of his second week in treatment neared, we discussed his next steps after leaving the hospital. His plan had been to transition to an inpatient residential program since he believed he was still vulnerable and needed to work more on his recovery in a relatively controlled setting. He requested a family meeting before his discharge. The plan was to have a family meeting before discharge. Donald's wife of 23 years, his son, and his sister came to the inpatient unit to bring him the warmth of winter clothes and loving support for the cold and challenging months ahead.

During the family meeting, Donald was able to express his realizations and understanding of his alcohol use and depression in a way that he never had been able to before. His sister, who had been in therapy for many years for her own struggle with depression, was thrilled to see her brother share what he had been going through for the first time. His wife who had been hurt emotionally and physically by Donald's addictive behaviors recognized the genuine change in him, though she was reluctant to be hopeful and vulnerable to being hurt by his behaviors yet again. She believed that, after years of trying to pick up the pieces and get him the help she knew he needed, she had to let go so he could figure it out for himself. She needed to care for herself and feared for the well-being of their son. Donald Jr. was torn as well, but was unable to give up on his father just yet. Tears fell from his face as he told his father, "I don't want to get my hopes up again, but regardless, alcohol will *never* stop me from loving you, Dad."

Donald reported feeling scared about moving on to his next phase of recovery. He was moved to tears as he expressed his gratitude for his experience working in treatment. He had grown to be more comfortable with opening up and had been surprised to learn how therapeutic and mobilizing sharing his stories had been for him. He expressed that he is a better person now and that he is on his way to reclaiming himself. Working with Donald made me realize the power of empathic listening.

What a rare and privileged profession it is in which a "day at work" consists of someone sharing the most intimate and painful details of their life *with* you. I was so fortunate to have the opportunity to be present with Donald and for all the lessons I have learned not just about addiction, depression, and losses but also about hope, humility, and resilience. Through the eyes of Donald, I experienced the deep emotional reality of suffering from alcohol use and depression, a sense of facing the stigma of addiction, and the healing impact of Zen listening and motivational interviewing.

Most importantly, I learned and cherished the value of allowing myself to be open and vulnerable to the raw emotions that come with sharing and listening in a genuine way. How incredible and fulfilling would it be if the MI and Zen practices were not solely a therapeutic approach but the norm with which we interact with each person we are so truly blessed to meet?

I built myself as a mindfulness-oriented psychiatrist through clinical training and practicing meditation and mindful listening. This is an ongoing learning process for me. I have realized that practicing mindfulness meditation did enhance my counseling skills such as empathy, acceptance, patience, genuineness, and positive regard. Furthermore, combined with my learning MI (MI spirit is defined as a *way of being* with patients), it strengthened my therapeutic presence with patients. Presence is defined as "an availability and openness to all aspects of the patient's experience, openness to one's own experience in being with the patient, and the capacity to respond to the patient from the experience" [7]. Siegel referred to the process as leading a patient to "feeling felt" [8]. Gendlin et al. [9] describe Rogers' concept of therapist genuineness as "being with the feelings and attitudes which at the moment are flowing within him" (p. 100). Practicing mindful listening and paying attention to my MI-inspired language have made my relationships with patients *real* and have considerably improved them. Evidently, it helped me feel and share a deeper genuineness and minimize my pseudo-empathic skills that contributed to burnout and detachment. I have, thus, become more capable of staying present and fully engaged in difficult therapeutic encounters without regressing, losing my empathy, and resorting to judgmental labeling (e.g., "He is an alcoholic and a big liar").

Surrey and Jordan [10] described *mutual empathy* as empathy being an ongoing relational process. The practitioner engages in the process of seeing and knowing by adapting and attuning to what the patient is experiencing. Empathy capitalizes on paying attention to a patient's body language, vocal tone, and other nonverbal cues, and, through the listening process and ongoing openness, synthesizing words, actions, and vocal cues until the patient feels heard, seen, and understood. The ultimate outcome is creating the experience of actually being accompanied through the journey of healing. In *The Healer's Power,* physician-scholar Howard Brody [11] coined the concept "empathic curiosity" to describe how being genuinely curious about patients' perspectives requires suspending judgment and allowing oneself to have some doubts. Empathy is promoted by cultivating curiosity that is grounded in an affective experience of connecting with the patient. Having a "curious and itchy mind" (as coined by Steve Rollnick) in practicing MI describes how listening to patients share more and tell their stories in their own words helps engender empathy.

Before I met Adam, all I knew about him was that he was a 40-year-old man who was admitted to the dual diagnosis unit after presenting to the emergency room with heavy daily heroin and alcohol use, increasing depression, and thoughts of "wanting to jump off a bridge or overdose on a bundle of heroin."

While working with him in treatment, one of the major themes Adam expressed was how he had used heroin in the past to control his negative emotions, particularly anger and rage. He shared that he had been "in and out, but mostly *in* jail" for the last 25 years, often for crimes of theft to support his use of heroin and alcohol. Adam soon disclosed more about his experiences in jail. He was constantly worried about his safety and joined the Aryan Brotherhood (also known as the "Brand," which is a white supremacist prison gang and organized crime syndicate in the US) for protection. He stated "I had to be angry all the time in case they needed me to fight or if someone tried to fight me," and that he used heroin to "smooth out those angry moods." He admitted he never disclosed to anyone before about his experiences in jail. He told me he felt "safe" to share them with me. From this conversation on, we developed a much deeper working relationship and I gradually gained a better understanding of his emotional struggles and the context of his substance use. Although I had no ability to relate in any way, shape, or form to his experiences in jail, I could certainly grasp through his sharing how the terrible fear and uncertainty about his safety led him to develop anger as a defensive tool. He told me that he never learned to regulate his emotions except by using drugs. He was very open to learning new coping strategies, including mindfulness-based approaches.

His newly learned coping skills for anger were challenged when Adam had an incident in the evening medication line. He became enraged at receiving a lower dose of diazepam than he had the day before. It had been previously discussed with him how the medication dose is tapered off over the course of few days to address his withdrawal from alcohol. His behavior escalated quickly and he became verbally abusive to the staff. To help him control his behavior and emotions, he was moved to a two-person room on the less stimulating wing of the unit. After Adam was moved to that wing, another patient was admitted to the unit and ended up being Adam's roommate. When Adam identified his roommate as African American, he became even angrier and started yelling racial slurs and intimidating the staff: "Don't you know that I'm in the Aryan Brotherhood?!" Eventually, Adam calmed down and declined an offer to be moved to a different room. Later, he went to his room with no further incident.

During our session the next day, I knew I had to address Adam's behaviors. I was overwhelmed, fearful, and confused, yet determined not to be overpowered by these emotions. Prior to the session, I attempted to refocus and practiced mindfulness to work through the intense emotions I was experiencing. By becoming mindful of the fear of being overwhelmed and scared, I became less intimidated and more confident to tackle the situation at hand. It was my turn to try to regulate my emotions. How was I going to explain the medication dosing without eliciting an angry reaction towards me? How would I address his anger towards his roommate and his racist beliefs that I did not share? I was ready to do it with an open mind. What I did was to attempt to normalize and validate his struggle with anger and how he was still working on regulating it by learning new ways, reemphasizing that it would be a process that takes time and hard work. I did not normalize his racist beliefs towards his roommate. I used empathic reflective listening and was able to maintain my composure. He was fully engaged with me and remained calm and respectful. We discussed his next steps for his recovery, and he had no further incidents with the medication regimen, his roommate, or the staff.

My experience working with Adam helped me gain greater perspective on the importance of empathy. I stayed *real* in my relationship with him. I shared with him that I struggled with understanding his gang experiences in prison and how they had shaped his beliefs about people of different race. At the same time, I expressed to him that I genuinely believed in his ability to change and validated his struggles with substance use as a means of soothing himself amidst powerful squalls of negative emotions. Through mindful listening and embracing the MI spirit, I was able to transform this challenging treatment experience full of mixed emotions into an opportunity to "be with" and "stay connected with" my patient. The equanimity cultivated in mindfulness practice and MI describes an attitude of open receptivity in which experience is welcomed. Through working with Adam, maintaining this evenness of mind taught me a lesson in humility and compassion and made me recognize the limits in my ability to change anyone other than myself.

References

1. Zuroff DC, Kelly AC, Leybman MJ, Blatt SJ, Wampold BE. Between-therapist and within-therapist differences in the quality of the therapeutic relationship: effects on maladjustment and self-critical perfectionism. J Clin Psychol. 2010;66(7):681–97.
2. Norcross JC, Wampold BE. Evidence-based therapy relationships: research conclusions and clinical practices. Psychotherapy (Chic). 2011;48(1):98–102.
3. Lown B. The lost art of healing: practicing compassion in medicine. New York: The Ballantine Publishing Group; 1996.
4. Suzuki S. Zen mind, beginner's mind. New York: Weatherhill; 1980.
5. Nhat Hanh T. Being peace. Berkley, CA: Parallax Press; 1987.
6. Blanche Hartman Z. Seeds for a boundless life: Zen teachings from the heart. Boston: Shambhala Publications, Inc.; 2015.
7. Geller SM, Greenberg LS. Therapeutic presence: therapists' experience of presence in the psychotherapy encounter. Person-Centered & Experiential Psychotherapies. 2002;1(1–2):71–86.

8. Siegel DJ. Emotion as integration: a possible answer to the question, what is emotion? In: Fosha D, Siegel DJ, Salomon M, editors. The healing power of emotion: affective neuroscience, development, and clinical practice. New York: W. W. Norton and Company; 2009. p. 145–71.
9. Rogers CR, Gendlin ET, Kiesler DJ, Truax CB, editors. The therapeutic relationship and its impact: a study of psychotherapy with schizophrenics. Madison, WI: University of Wisconsin Press; 1967. p. 73–93.
10. Surrey J, Jordan JV. The wisdom of connection. In: Germer CK, Siegel DJ, editors. Wisdom and compassion in psychotherapy: deepening mindfulness in clinical practice. New York: Guilford Press; 2002. p. 163–75.
11. Brody H. The Healer's power. New Haven and London: Yale University Press; 1992.

Chapter 3
Learning and Growing from Unpredictable Encounters

> *"Always be drunk. That's it--that's all that matters. So you won't feel the horrible burden of Time which breaks your shoulder and bends you to the ground, you need to get drunk without end.*
> *But with what? With wine, poetry or virtue--it's your choice. But get drunk. And if sometime--on the steps of a palace, on the green grass of a gulley, in the somber solitude of your room--you wake up, the drunkenness already diminished or gone; then ask the wind, the wave, the star, the bird, all that runs away, all that groans, all that rolls, all that sings, all that talks--ask them what time it is; and the wind, the wave, the star, the bird, the clock will answer you: 'It's time to get drunk! So you won't be martyred slaves of Time: get drunk, get drunk without end. With wine, poetry, or virtue--it's your choice.'"*
>
> —Charles Baudelaire: "Enivrez-vous" ("Get Drunk") from Le Spleen de Paris

No matter how much experience and knowledge I might have, I continually question what I do in my clinical work. This perpetual questioning keeps my mind open. It keeps me open to understanding myself and my patients. It keeps me in my "Zen mind, beginner's mind." Along the same line, I have questioned what it means for me to be "helpful and make a difference" in treatment. I wonder what my role is in the "helping relationship" and how it fits in with practicing what we know "scientifically" to produce a positive outcome with our patients. I admit that I have often lapsed into believing that, if I *just* practice evidence-based treatments, my patients *should* do better. In fact, I have the full evidence from my clinical life that what can turn out to be helpful and mobilizing for the patient's recovery from addiction is not necessarily that which I had thought of as likely to do it. Sometimes, the most healing of therapeutic elements in the most unexpected of moments have not been gathered from any study but from the interpersonal chemistry that can occur only in the most human of encounters.

I recall from my psychodynamic training in residency the immense focus on how much the therapists' characteristics affect their work: the therapists' "values, assumptions, and psychological idiosyncrasies" [1]; their "own dynamic, passions, ideas, and general subjectivity" [2]; and their "experiences and personal development "[3]. Clearly, so many factors can influence the clinical outcomes, before we even consider the patient's contributions! Working through defining my own theoretical orientation and identity, I have realized that what best defines me in my clinical work is being mindfully open-minded when I am with patients. This kind of "knowing naiveté," as I once thought of it, is best captured by a beloved English novelist who calls it being "woolly-minded":

> "*It is the woolly mind that combines skepticism of everything with credulity about everything. Being woolly has no hard edges. It is easy, pliant, yet it has its own toughness. Because it bends, it does not break... The woolly mind realizes that we live in an unimaginable gigantic, complicated, mysterious universe. To try to stuff the vast bewildering creation into a few neat pigeon-holes is absurd. We do not know enough, and to pretend we do is mere intellectual conceit. (Almost all men who like to refer scornfully to woolly minds suffer from this conceit.) The best we can do is to keep looking out for clues, for anything that will light up a step or two into the dark... The woolly mind can be silly at times, but even so, it finds out more and enjoys more than the rat-trap intelligence. Second-rate scientists are never woolly minded where as great scientists let their minds go woolly between experiments*." ([4]; J. B. Priestley, 1972, 30–1).

The concept of "subjectivity" in clinical work is fascinating for many reasons, not only because it is such a necessary element in healing, but also because it is so exclusive of the "objectivity" that is supposed to inform our extrapolation from, say, the scientific literature to our clinical work. It is often confused or connected with countertransference. Clearly, our own human—and deeply personal—reactions to *each patient* are expected, inevitable, and should not be viewed as inherently problematic [5]. Our own personal reactions can be deeply informative and have a major impact on our patients. They represent who we are as therapists and human beings; they are the stuff of a healing encounter itself. Avoiding and minimizing our own subjectivity compromises our "authenticity" and can distance us from our patients' most important experiences, when it is emotional attunement and presence that are most therapeutically necessary. Being forthcoming about our reactions to ourselves and each other makes the clinical encounter more real and gives our patients the ability to deal with our subjectivity more openly [1]. Trying to balance being emotionally intimate with a patient and yet separate is my own most ongoing challenge. It is one that I deal with frequently in external supervision but in each moment with my own "internalized supervision" [6]. This latter supervision was defined by Casement as a therapist's "capacity to function with more immediate (but not instant) *insight* within the momentum of the therapeutic process."

The following clinical stories illustrate the challenges in establishing and sustaining a therapeutic relationship with patients in unpredictable encounters. They also reveal how I strive to intertwine my own subjectivity with my scientific approach. In these encounters, I share my struggle to accept my own limitations as I learn that healing and growth ultimately emerge from both the scientific and humanistic dilemmas of the encounter.

Our team could easily tell the atmosphere on the dual diagnosis unit was so tense and loaded with judgmental attitudes. During the morning report, staff members were talking in hushed voices about Lisa, a patient who was just admitted to the unit. Apparently, Lisa managed to sneak heroin into the unit and one of the nurses found her with a syringe in her arm the previous night. I was so furious at how staff had allowed a major breach of safety: Lisa could have easily overdosed and died on the very unit that was supposed to help her! Furthermore, what she did jeopardized the safety of all patients on the unit. Following our policy of zero tolerance for drugs on the unit, we were quickly, perhaps reactively, moved to discharge her from the unit immediately due to her behaviors. But swift discharge was not an option. Her case was typical but in key ways unique. She was homeless. She had no support system. She had a total laryngectomy for a highly advanced throat cancer which left her voiceless. The same condition also left her nutritionally dependent on a feeding tube. Discharging her to the street was not an option after all. We had little choice but to rethink how to approach her care on the unit. We reluctantly turned our focus to her reckless drug taking behaviors and need for long-term placement.

For the first few days, Lisa refused to engage in treatment and secluded herself in her room. Her social withdrawal was extremely frustrating for our team. A medical student stepped forward to work with Lisa on a one-on-one basis since she was not engaged in our daily team rounds. The medical student expressed that "something about her tugged me into her issues, and looking back, I think it was partly out of fear that she would be overlooked and discharged before giving her a chance to get started with her recovery." Lisa continued to refuse to share her struggles despite the medical student's efforts to make engagement safe and open. She stayed present with the patient even though she barely said (or wrote) anything. The medical student described feeling *insecure, foolish, unprofessional, and helpless*. However, she expressed to the team: *I could tell she was listening to me*.

The next day, the patient joined our team for the first time. Until that point, most of our work with Lisa was focused on addressing her complicated medical issues and safe housing options- after all that was what she insisted on! But was that our immediate focus?

In Lisa's case, it was clear to me that we had to mind the utilization of different interventions within a greater scope. Every day when considering her treatment, we had in mind that the most effective treatment approaches for substance use disorders do not focus necessarily or exclusively on the addiction itself, but also emphasize the importance of general coping skills and quality of life [7, 8], as well as focus on solving social problems of housing and basic life needs. Following such an interdisciplinary collaborative therapeutic approach, the whole team was mobilized to assist Lisa, utilizing case management and behavioral therapy in lieu of pharmacological interventions.

Our work with Lisa crystallized for me the role of *engagement* and *alliance*. Alliance seemed non-existent initially as Lisa maintained a distance after her egregious drug use behavior on the unit. It was only through the consistent, empathic engagement of a dedicated medical student sharing the motivational spirit that finally led our team to realize that this voiceless patient was listening during their encounters. The other treatments and care strategies that we would deploy to help Lisa might have been nullified without having first striven for engagement and alliance in a motivational way. Lisa put our clinical services into perspective. I came to view the empirically-based addiction treatments at our disposal as the bricks that are necessary for a solid treatment plan. However, it is the humanistic and motivational engagement—which I consider to be almost a spiritual art—that is the mortar that not only brings the treatment plan together as one but also binds the therapeutic dyad into a collaborative whole.

Working with Lisa was very challenging in part because of how unpredictable it was. For one thing, her ability to deal with strong emotions was so limited, as she initially expressed that she was looking for housing and nothing else. During her first week on the unit, she went through a drastic change in her thinking and motivation to change because after a few sessions she started to express that she wanted to stop using heroin and was willing to do whatever it would take to reclaim herself and attain recovery. The team was so optimistic and hopeful that she could make it. Clearly, we knew it was not an easy road to recovery. Reviewing her support network, she shared that some family members were active users of drugs. She said further that she was not willing to cut ties with them even though initially she did not identify them as a part of her support system. She was fiercely protective of them and struggled to acknowledge their potential negative impact on her recovery. She shared that she had few things in her life that she felt worth living for, and the main one was *her family*. From her concerns, we reasoned that we had to respect her autonomy and adjust our expectations to match hers: *we had to meet her where she was in her journey.*

In our final session with her, she expressed her gratitude to the medical student and the whole team. We felt as a team that we had woven together the most important biopsychosocial threads to wrap her up in a strong discharge plan. Empirically, we *know* that patients who are involved with medical and social services are likely to remain longer in addiction treatment and tend to have better outcomes in terms of psychological well-being and reduced substance use compared to people who do not receive such services [9, 10]. We used this knowledge to create a strong discharge plan which included coordinated medical and social services as well as a referral to an addiction treatment program. But we only achieved this collaboratively-derived plan by working so diligently to improve the quality of our interactions with Lisa!

Working with Lisa was an intense and powerful experience. Emotionally, I was deeply challenged and sometimes doubted how much I had "left in the tank" to continue to engage her empathically and without judgment. After our work with Lisa, it was the medical student who had found the words that I alone had not been able to find myself:

> "*While working with Lisa, I was constantly worried that I might have been able to do more for her, and that what I did would not be enough to help her to reach her recovery. At times, I felt confused, and found myself wondering if I truly was making a difference with her. However, I do feel confident that my experience with her will continue to inspire me to connect with patients for the rest of my career in medicine.*"

These words echoed my deepest feelings and spoke for the collective experience that we had together as a treatment team.

One of my finest teachers was Mary who gave herself and me the opportunity to learn to trust and test out how best to establish a working relationship. Mary presented for treatment of severe depression and alcohol use disorder. Initially, she described feeling severely depressed, lonely, hopeless, and ashamed of her drinking and its impact on her life and her family. She had been trying to control her addiction to alcohol for years, as she felt it had cost her dearly, including the life she thought she could have and connections she needed most. At that point in her treatment, she felt able to talk about these decisions and losses in a way she had not known was possible. She struggled through these deep emotional issues she had delayed dealing with for so long as she scrutinized her own inability to commit to sobriety previously. Yet, she focused poignantly on her recovery, gaining a new perspective on her addiction to alcohol as serving to self-soothe deep, longstanding feelings of grief, shame, and guilt. Mary became very open as she fully immersed herself in treatment: she participated in groups, completed interactive workbooks, and journaled about her struggles with depression and alcohol use. My work with her sought to integrate all the objective knowledge that I had about addiction treatment while also using my own subjectivity to connect with Mary on the most human of levels. I focused on strengthening her motivation for change, redefining her value system, teaching her coping skills and other relapse prevention strategies, addressing emotional regulation, integrating care of her dual disorders, identifying more social resources in the community, establishing case management services, and optimizing her medication regimen.

Mary had been treated in drug rehabilitation programs in the past, but it was evident to both of us that this moment in her life was different. She strongly believed she was confident to pursue intensive outpatient treatment post discharge. She described her current treatment experience as "empowering her." She described an "epiphany" after which she felt a sense of inner peace and commitment to a better life and self. As she was discharged on a Friday afternoon, I shared with her a sense of hopefulness for her continued journey of recovery as I believed she would fare well.

On the following Monday morning, we performed our routine check on recently discharged patients and whether they followed up at their scheduled post-discharge appointments. I was so disappointed, angry, and demoralized to learn that Mary had been seen the day before in the emergency room of a different hospital for breathing problems and had a very high blood alcohol level.

"What did I do wrong?" I simmered to myself. Did I fail the patient? What clues about her struggles did I miss?

My initial anger was mixed with questions and second guessing; I did not know if I was blaming myself or the patient. I was wracked with self-doubt. I questioned whether she was genuine in her investment in recovery. I debated through my "internalized supervision" whether I should have encouraged her to consider a residential program; maybe that would have changed the outcome. I had moments of feeling responsible myself for her drinking after discharge. I also found it within me to try to listen, observe, and maybe learn from these inner voices of doubt and frustration; in that moment it was so hard for me to do the deep reflection that was of course necessary to find meaning in this painful experience. I realized that I had to do exactly what I wanted Mary to do for herself during our work together: to find ways to regulate her powerful feelings by learning to notice and process them so she could find her own meaning in what was otherwise the chaotic internal milieu that made her so vulnerable to using alcohol in the first place. As I strained to look within myself, my thinking then turned towards what it might have been like for Mary and how she might have felt before and after her use of alcohol so soon after leaving treatment. She must have again gone through overwhelming feelings of shame and despair. It must have been a repetition of the same feelings and urges to deal with those feelings that she had shared openly but with difficulty only days before. She had tried so hard recently and in the past to overcome her addiction and cope with her depression; of course, part of my thinking about her must mean recognizing her history of vulnerability to her emotional difficulties and to relapse itself.

In my own fantasy, I had hoped that her experience with me would be the one to get her started on her recovery journey. In fact, this was the reason I was trying to help her build connections to a support system to reduce setbacks in her recovery. In thinking about her recent lapse, I hoped her drinking behavior after discharge to be an isolated episode that she could learn from to refocus on her recovery. I noticed myself wishing that her last treatment episode would decrease the number and severity of these episodes. In this deeply emotional reverie, I reflected on a thorny question that had long chafed me since I had first started studying the scientific literature on addiction. I struggled with the black-or-white thinking about addiction outcomes that is inherent in the concept of "relapse" itself. Of course, we are familiar with the long held idea that a major goal in the management of chronic medical illnesses including addiction is to extend spans of remission and to reduce the length and severity of symptomatic episodes [11]. I had to find within this scientific fact a new personal meaning where before I had been prone to think of relapse as some kind of failure, and in this case I thought it was my own failure! Maybe Mary had a "lapse" which did not mean "relapse"? How would I know for sure whether her treatment with me did not impact her in a meaningful way? Good time for the Serenity Prayer! I found myself striving to find hope and meaning in what I initially experienced as futility and failure. Through these internal fumblings over what this episode was about, I found what I wanted Mary to find in herself: that she can notice and find the meaning in her own vulnerabilities and fallibilities as a process of learning about herself the same way I did as I reflected on how this experience with her changed me in a deeper emotional way.

As I have grown as an addiction psychiatrist, I have believed more firmly in the impact of evidence-based treatments. It has been awe-inspiring to have seen firsthand the transformations patients can undergo throughout the process of treatment. The most carefully constructed studies and trials show with confidence that our treatments work on a macro-scale. It is something else entirely to see them "work" in the life of a person. It is astonishing to see the power of these treatments as pieces in the transformative work of recovery.

Working with James had a significant impact on me even though his treatment experience did not "transform" him! James was a man in his late 20s with a history of polysubstance use. His drug of choice was heroin. He had multiple treatment episodes on our dual diagnosis unit and was well known to our staff, often evoking powerful negative reactions in those therapists who worked most closely with him. They referred to him as a "manipulator and drug seeker." During the morning report, several staff members rolled their eyes and exchanged looks that implied, "let's see how long before he signs out against medical advice (AMA) this time." I welled up with anger as I strained to stay composed stopping just short of castigating the staff. I sought a moment of mindfulness and tried to maintain whatever mental focus I had for the patient himself.

Our encounter with him during the treatment team rounds was brief since he stated he was going through withdrawal. He made poor eye contact with me, repeatedly insisting "I know what I need to do. Right now, I just need to detox here." He was willing to share nothing else but his desire for medical attention to his withdrawal symptoms. It was only hours later that day that he did decide to leave by signing out AMA. We tried to engage him, but he refused to negotiate about further treatment, even for a short duration. Denying that he had any expectations from treatment, he insisted on leaving immediately. I felt defeated. The efforts at connection with him as well as my energy to contain my frustrations at the cynicism during our treatment team meeting that morning left me feeling all was for naught. A staff member even reminded me "we told you so!" I struggled against feelings of depletion as I once again re-centered myself through mindfulness and sought to find meaning in my continued belief in the work I do with patients and in their ability to change. I searched within myself for the motivational spirit; I needed to ferret out whatever I could of those collaborative and compassionate aspects of that spirit by which I could give James the benefit of the doubt and find within him (as I sought within myself!) the proverbial "better angels of our nature."

Just as I was struggling to accept the limitations I was feeling with myself, I accepted that James was not ready to change *now* and hoped that the next time in treatment he would consider addressing his addiction. A week later, when it was announced that James had been readmitted, the staff's cynicism reached a new pitch: "He's just back because he couldn't get any more dope on the street"; "He will not get *any* detoxification medication this time and particularly buprenorphine!" Boiling inside, I was again challenged to contain the strong urge I had to respond in anger to these statements. Again, I refocused my energy on James and the mission in caring for patients which I knew was the reason why I and even our wary staff continued to do this work. I held fast to the hope that he would engage in treatment this time and that I could be part of evoking from him just a step or two on the journey of recovery.

During the treatment team rounds, he appeared deeply ill with all the clinical stigmata of a severe withdrawal syndrome. However, he also appeared to be different compared to his presentation only weeks ago. Though he was hunched over, rocking in his chair, and clutching himself across his belly, he mustered some attentiveness to our being together. He neither slouched nor sloughed off any part of our session this time. I was astonished at the way he shared himself to the point of virtual free association.

James stated starkly that he had overdosed four times since his discharge. He frankly stated that "I know all about" the treatment programs; it was clear he was involved in some of them though to an unclear extent. As far as James could tell, however, the degree of his involvement in treatment was not the point. He was deeply emotionally perplexed at himself: he kept using and could not figure out why he was so "self-destructive" and dominated by his addiction. He felt stuck and had long believed that dying was the only way out of this vicious cycle. Finding no reason or idea within himself for which to continue living, he expressed that his father and sister were the only people who stopped him from ending it all; he even expressed aloud his wish that they would stop caring.

The atmosphere in the rounding room took on an emotional weight I had not yet known as he made clear in the plainest of words a misery and despair he had lived with throughout most of his life. To me and the team, it made total sense why he totally dismissed treatment and claimed to know all about it. At that moment, we felt the pain that had been experienced by him but was not yet verbalized; and it was a pain which, while mostly unspoken, certainly had not yet been witnessed or understood by another. We spoke privately about our own doubts about being able to help him as we sought to shrink from the emotional burdens he had been bearing and was now sharing with us. I doubted my own clinical and emotional wherewithal to help him. His sense of hopelessness shook our collective belief in treatment. We felt guilty for our low expectations, heartbroken on his behalf, and at the same time we tried hard to sustain hopefulness and drive to do whatever we could to help him work through this excruciating moment in his journey. We thought his first step of sharing could be a breakthrough in the process of recovery. Our optimism and hope lasted for a few days until he signed out AMA after a long weekend. Again, he was not willing to negotiate remaining in treatment and would not acknowledge his vulnerability in view of the premature discharge that he was choosing.

We realized our team went through a traumatic experience. We were confused and angry. Reaching out for help was already so painful for him, and we had assumed the worst in him. How could he have not noticed our reactions and feelings towards him? How could we have not noticed that it was perhaps our own attitudes at the outset which might have been the impediments to having a more fulfilling care relationship with James than the one we ultimately had, the one which left him discontinuing treatment and us questioning our roles as healthcare practitioners? Did we undermine our own work by not recognizing how we might have imposed our own expectations about his recovery on him? Did we do this at the expense of understanding him and where he was in his recovery? I reflected more deeply on the staff's low expectations of him and lack of empathy towards him. Instead, they were protecting themselves from being disappointed repeatedly as they detached themselves from him and were not willing to accept him for who he was or where he was in his journey. I believe that, in their own way of protecting their own vulnerability to disappointment, they dismissed him. His signing to leave AMA felt like a broken care relationship, which to a devoted professional, is among the most hurtful of experiences. I viewed their approach as counter-therapeutic and harmful to the patient. It demonstrated exactly what I do not want to do with my patients; it was antithetical to how I saw myself as a healer. Yes, I realize that I should take a certain "distance" from the patient, and yet I also need and want to be present, empathic, and in touch with my own and the patient's feelings and reactions. I had long seen these elements as ingredients in the recipe of healing, but they were missing in this experience with James.

Low level of empathy in addiction treatment can be considered toxic, as research has shown that patients whose practitioners show low levels of accurate empathy have particularly poor outcomes relative to patients working with high-empathy practitioners [12]. The authors' conclusion confirmed a clinical intuition I had long harbored within me. As one of my mentors expressed, "we don't take credits for the change our patients make nor do we blame ourselves for the change they did not make." This wisdom has been so sparing for me in my work with patients. I know the ways in which I must be present to help the process of a patient's recovery. I also have to recognize the limits I have in the caring therapeutic relationship: though I strive to be a caring presence in working with a patient towards recovery, I can own no part of the patient's journey, and, in this way, I can own no part of a patient's lapses. I am not implying to simply take a "neutral supporter" role in the helping relationship; far from it. What I mean is that embracing this perspective allows one to be more actively engaged in a more healing way with the patient rather than being overly invested in a way that can make one vulnerable to the very disappointment and hardness to which I believe our staff fell prey in this broken care episode with James. I wonder how things might have been different if we could start over by engaging with James in a more empathic way and focusing on setting goals and building personal strengths (Cognitive-Based Therapy with Recovery focus, as called by Aaron Beck). I wonder if we then would have experienced with James openness or vulnerability that was clearly every bit as difficult for him as it was for us.

The mutual empathy [13] which was not so clearly present in this episode with James is deeply central to the healing process in the therapeutic relationship. Jordan [13] describes relational processes that foster growth and transformation in relational-cultural therapy:

> *"A model that recognizes that therapy is a dialogue also recognizes that therapy is characterized by a process of mutual change and impact. Both therapist and patient are touched emotionally by each other, grow in relationship, gain something from one another, risk something of themselves in the process... In short, both are affected, changed, part of an open system of feeling and learning. There is significant mutuality. It takes courage on both sides to involve themselves in this interaction."*

Each patient story is unique. At the same time, there are common themes that can be found in almost all stories. Perhaps the most ubiquitous of these themes is deep emotional pain. For Tom, the pain started early. He was just a toddler when his father shook him so hard that his lungs collapsed. By the time he was 10 years old, he had been diagnosed with depression. He began to see a therapist and was prescribed various antidepressants. At that time, he reports receiving support from his step-father, who introduced him to motocross racing. The patient competed in these events across the country with some success. Then he suffered an injury in a racing accident that resulted in back surgeries and left him with debilitating chronic pain. It was then that he was exposed to opioids. His subsequent path was characterized by his own misuse as well as some instances of iatrogenic dependence. He became powerfully addicted to them. His struggle with depression continued through the age of 20 when he was hospitalized for attempted overdose on alcohol and bupropion. Several years later, his addiction progressed to heroin. Gradually, his use destroyed his relationships and his career. Desperate, he enrolled in a rehabilitation program after which he maintained sobriety for a year until his step-father committed suicide after which he started using again. Eighteen months later, he presented to the hospital for treatment reporting severe addiction to opioids, deep depression, and hopelessness.

When I and our team first met Tom, he was in severe opioid withdrawal. Despite his symptoms, he was still attentive, articulate, and expressed his commitment to stop using and work towards his recovery. He appeared to have insight into the nature of his addiction, the suffering it had brought upon him and the ones he loved, and the necessary steps to achieve and maintain recovery. During the second person-centered MI-focused session, I asked the patient about his relationship with his step-father and the impact of his suicide. At first, the patient was reluctant to share, but eventually he disclosed and cried. He divulged a deep sadness, anger, and sense of abandonment he felt in the wake of the event. He also acknowledged that his use was in part a means of evading the unbearable pain he felt at the time. At the end of the session, he revealed that this was the first time he had re-experienced "feelings of loss" since his step-father's funeral 18 months ago. I left for the weekend hopeful that Tom would continue to engage not only in the detoxification process, but also in addressing the painful emotions that had been contributing to his longstanding use.

Upon returning to the unit on Monday morning, I was surprised to learn that Tom had decided to leave AMA. When I asked him about his decision he told us that he felt there was nothing more to be gained from inpatient treatment. Now that he was done with withdrawal, he was eager to return home and continue his recovery in an outpatient treatment program. He reported that morning that he was feeling "great," as it became apparent that he was no longer willing to share his emotions with us. We approached him to see if he would consider involving his mother and sister in his treatment by having a family meeting, but he was adamantly opposed to this suggestion. He insisted that the issues he wanted to work out with them would be best worked out "privately." Both his mother and girlfriend had requested to visit him on the unit but he had refused. He informed us that he had kept his heroin addiction *a secret* from his girlfriend, telling her instead that he was addicted to Suboxone® (Indivior, Richmond, VA, USA). We asked him how he felt his girlfriend would respond when she found out about his heroin addiction and that he had lied to her. He replied that she would either accept him or reject him, and if she were to leave him he would simply move on and find another woman.

Initially, we thought his flippant response was merely a defensive move devised to avoid facing the shame related to his addictive behaviors and the pain of potentially losing his girlfriend. As he engaged more, however, it seemed he had not fully come to grips with the immense pain he was causing his loved ones. Whether he was unaware of the consequences of his actions or simply refused to acknowledge them was not clear. Regardless, it was frustrating and demoralizing for me to witness him share the week before only to shut me and the team out the following week. It was also surprising to me because when he had first arrived he expressed that he was willing to do whatever it would take to be successful in his recovery. By the second week, however, his position was to "detox and leave." Perhaps that was his intention from the beginning, or perhaps he experienced *something* when he shared that he wasn't willing to continue tapping into. I wonder if those "feelings of loss" which had long been unexperienced were as scary as they were painful for him. I wondered if instead of helping him have deeper emotional clarity that they instead were bewildering for him. I wondered if his flight from the hospital was also a flight from the scene of these long suppressed feelings.

During our final session, I shared with Tom that recovery is more than detoxing and avoiding relapse, that it also involves engaging in the pain, emotions, and patterns of thinking that contribute to the use and learning to deal with these phenomena in a healthy manner and ultimately reclaim himself. Recovery also incorporates acknowledging the consequences one's addiction has had on family and friends, and engaging in the hard work of reconciliation and rebuilding trust. He listened but did not seem to process what we tried to impart. He seemed so disconnected. Then it hit me. In that moment, I experienced within me the deeper truth of a long held aphorism in the field: the opposite of addiction is connection. This disconnectedness that I was experiencing with Tom at that point was so frustrating for me! I felt thwarted and ineffective! I realized that this could be akin to what Tom could have been experiencing within himself ever since these losses and abandonments early in his own life. People do not become addicted in a vacuum, I thought. Nor do people with addiction recover in a vacuum. At that point, Tom was still making his way in a vacuum of his own experience where connections were painfully lost and the prospect of new ones triggered the experience of buried pains that threatened to overwhelm him. So, of course Tom's choice to continue addressing his addiction and maintain his distance from caring people in his life made sense to me. Yes, to me the opposite of addiction still meant connection; but connection for Tom was anything but safe.

Most recoveries happen without any professional help. It is humbling to realize that we can rarely feel so confident in making any prediction about a patient's individual outcome from treatment even if we know that treatment works. The impact of therapeutic work on our patients' lives is unpredictable. We play a relatively momentary and minor therapeutic role in the struggles of our patients' lives. David Treadway [14] likened therapy to *Hamlet's* Rosencrantz and Guildenstern; we arrive in the middle of the play, have our lines, do our turn, but rarely get to see the ending. In some cases, patients might begin their story like the play's dejected adolescent-like protagonist (and namesake) who struggles to be truthful with himself and those around him about his deepest conflicts. We cannot be certain which of our patients will go on like Hamlet to find the courage to take responsibility for himself, his mistakes, and fate. What we can do, however, is to stay devoted to playing our best therapeutic role in the scene in which we enter into that patient's story. Our best role might mean being nothing more than absolutely present and attentive to the words and emotions of the patient's own internal drama while the patient struggles forward to own them and her behaviors, addictive and otherwise. What a profound experience it is to walk together through *pain* with a patient who comes to us with emotional injuries seeking to be understood and accepted for who she is! Equally humbling is recognizing that for as much as we might work to help the patient, our efforts are so miniscule compared to the heroics of the patient in overcoming struggles that we might not even see after we have done our best to play our part.

References

1. Renik O. Analytic interaction: conceptualizing technique in light of the analyst's irreducible subjectivity. Psychoanal Q. 1993;62:553–71.
2. Mitchell SA, Black M. Freud and beyond: a history of modern psychoanalytic thought. New York: Basic Books; 1995.
3. Winnicott DW. Hate in the counter-transference. Int J Psychoanal. 1994;3(4):348–56.
4. Casement P. Learning from the patient. New York: Guilford Press; 1991.
5. Hoffman IZ. Dialectical thinking and therapeutic action in the psychoanalytic process. Psychoanal Q. 1994;63:187–218.
6. Casement P. Learning from our mistakes: beyond dogma and psychotherapy. New York: Guilford Press; 2002.
7. Miller WR, Carroll KM. Rethinking substance abuse. Motivational factors in addictive behaviors. In: Miller WR, Carroll KM, editors. Rethinking substance abuse. New York: Guilford Press; 2006. p. 134–52.
8. Miller WR, Wilbourne PL, Hettema JE. What works? A summary of alcohol treatment outcome research. In: Hester RK, Miller WR, editors. Handbook of alcoholism treatment approaches: effective alternatives. 3rd ed. Boston: Allyn and Bacon; 2003. p. 13–63.
9. Hesse M, Vanderplasschen W, Rapp RC, Broekaert E, Fridell M. Case management for persons with substance use disorders. Cochrane Database Syst Rev. 2007;(4):CD006265.
10. Morgenstern J, Hogue A, Dauber S, Dasaro C, McKay JR. A practical clinical trial of coordinated care management to treat substance use disorders among public assistance beneficiaries. J Consult Clin Psychol. 2009;77(2):257–69.
11. Miller WR, Westerberg VS, Harris RJ, Tonigan JS. What predicts relapse? Prospective testing of antecedent models. Addiction. 1996;91(Suppl):S155–71.
12. Moyers TB, Miller WR. Is low therapist empathy toxic? Psychol Addict Behav. 2013;27(3):878–84.
13. Jordan JV. The role of mutual empathy in relational/cultural therapy. J Clin Psychol. 2000;56(8):1005–16.
14. Treadway DC. Intimacy, change, and other therapeutic mysteries: stories of clinicians and clients. New York: Guilford Press; 2004.

Part II
On Integrating Science and Humanistic Practice

> *"The most beautiful experience we can have is the mysterious. It is the fundamental emotion which stands at the cradle of true art and true science. Whoever does not know it and can no longer wonder, no longer marvel, is as good as dead, and his eyes are dimmed .... A knowledge of the existence of something we cannot penetrate, our perceptions of the profoundest reason and the most radiant beauty, which only in their most primitive forms are accessible to our minds--it is this knowledge and this emotion that constitute true religiosity; in this sense, and in this alone, I am a deeply religious man."*
>
> —Albert Einstein: The World as I See It, 1935: 24–28

Part II explores what may arguably be the most challenging aspect of practicing addiction medicine-integrating humanism and science. This section provides conceptual frameworks for understanding addiction and its treatment approaches. It argues for the importance of practicing pragmatically with an open mind, selecting scientifically-informed therapeutic modalities, and respecting the patient's collaborative involvement in the therapeutic process. I share clinical stories that highlight the importance of a dialectical interplay between science and humanism: integrating scientific facts with a philosophy that values the uniqueness of each story and the spirit of collaboration in the journey towards healing.

Chapter 4
Scientific Foundations for Addiction Practice

> *"Why are you drinking? - The little prince asked. - In order to forget - replied the drunkard. - To forget what? - inquired the little prince, who was already feeling sorry for him.*
> *- To forget that I am ashamed - the drunkard confessed, hanging his head. - Ashamed of what? - asked the little prince who wanted to help him. - Ashamed of drinking! - concluded the drunkard, withdrawing into total silence. And the little prince went away, puzzled. 'Grown-ups really are very, very odd', he said to himself as he continued his journey."*
>
> —Antoine de Saint-Exupéry: The Little Prince

Introduction

While writing this chapter, I debated and brainstormed about the best way to share the science of addiction and differentiate clearly opinion from scientific finding. I realized that I wanted to avoid overloading the readers with a lot of data and instead plan to provide a simple, clear, practical, and succinct summary and discussion of the interrelationships among research data findings and their implications for clinical practice. This chapter is my best distillation of how current scientific discoveries could make a significant impact on alleviating the personal suffering and reducing the societal costs related to the addictive disorders. My personal experiences are shared throughout this scientific journey. Furthermore, I avoided as much as possible making recommendations for any specific approaches and focused more on principles and concepts that need to be integrated into our systems of care and our bigger societal response to the substance use problems. As I gained experience and practice in addiction treatment, my challenge was to confront my own biases and misperceptions and keep an open mind, realizing that I still have so much to learn and deal with unresolved scientific puzzles. I hope you will take the same approach.

The field of addiction has evolved dramatically in the last three decades. How far have we progressed because of the scientific knowledge? Do we have a shared vision on how we approach, understand, and treat addictions? What are the challenges that we continue to encounter in the diffusion of innovations into clinical practice? And how can we address public skepticism that remains so strong at a time when scientific progress has been growing significantly?

Historical Context and Theoretical Models of Addiction

The U.S. temperance movement, which originally advocated for moderation in the use of alcohol, became a prohibition movement in 1920. The 18th Amendment to the U.S. Constitution was ratified, making it illegal to manufacture, sell, transport, or import "intoxicating liquor." At that time, alcohol was considered as a medically and socially dangerous drug, and drinkers were considered capable of inflicting great harm on society. It was also understood that alcohol could not be used for long in moderation and that people who drink are headed for insanity and death. The only choice was abstinence. The 18th Amendment was repealed by the 21st Amendment in 1933. The "war on drugs" of the late twentieth century is a typical example of blaming the "agent" (the drug itself) with the only remedy being to eliminate the drug from the society. In 1935, the Alcoholics Anonymous (AA) movement was formed as a solution to help people recover from "alcoholism." It emphasized that only *certain* people are at risk for "alcoholism," that "alcoholics" are different from normal people, and that "non-alcoholics" can drink with impunity. The large scientific literature on mutual support programs, particularly AA, will be described later in the book.

The American Psychiatric Association's *Diagnostic and Statistical Manual of Mental Disorders* (DSM) [1] has been the standard for classification by behavioral health providers in North America as the framework for the conceptualization of addictive disorders. The DSM provides specific diagnoses that fit a person's clinical presentation. The diagnostic approach is binary—present or absent—even though practice and research show one size fits all is not a reality and people are more on a continuum. In the early 1950s, the first edition of the DSM (DSM-I) [1] came out putting both *alcoholism and drug addiction* in the same category of sociopathic personality disturbances, implying that people with addiction suffered from "deep seated personality disturbance." In the same category, they also included sexual deviations and antisocial behavior, indicating that people with addictions were dangerous to society. In addition, the DSM-I identified addiction as a manifestation of an underlying brain or personality disorder with no specific details of the symptoms and signs exhibited by the individual with an addiction!

In the second edition of the DSM (DSM-II, 1968) [2], new terms were introduced to describe different types of "alcoholism" such as *episodic excessive drinking, habitual excessive drinking,* and *alcohol addiction*. These descriptions fit *the Disease Concept of Alcoholism* introduced by Jellinek [3]. *Drug dependence* was also detailed in the DSM-II to include subcategories by specific drug class. As in the DSM-I, these disorders remained under the same rubric of "personality disorders and certain other non-psychotic mental disorders."

The DSM-III (1980) [4] included the first classification to separate substance abuse and substance dependence from other categories such as personality disorders. Longitudinal research clearly indicated that many individuals with a history of alcohol use never progress to a full-blown dependence level. "Alcoholism" was dropped as a formal diagnosis. The DSM-III did not delineate any specific etiologies to substance abuse and dependence, and attempted to move away from conceptualizing addiction as a personal pathology. *Substance abuse* was defined as problematic use with social and/or occupational impairment, but with the absence of tolerance (the need to take higher doses of the substance to have the same effect) and/or withdrawal syndrome (physiological changes after stopping or reducing the use of substance). *Substance dependence* was defined by the physiological symptoms of tolerance and withdrawal, and required the presence of either one or both criteria in addition to social and occupational impairment.

The DSM-III was revised in 1987 (DSM-III-R) [5] and emphasized a similar importance of both the behavioral and physiological aspects of substance use disorders. The DSM-III-R category of psychoactive substance abuse was identified as a pattern of use that continues despite awareness of negative consequences or by drug use in situations in which it is physically dangerous.

The DSM-IV (1994) [6] continued with similar categories of abuse and dependence. It also included other diagnoses concerned with drug-related intoxication: withdrawal, delirium, mood disorders, anxiety disorders, etc. The criteria for abuse and dependence were separated in the DSM-IV. Dependence was defined as a syndrome involving compulsive use, with or without tolerance, and withdrawal. Abuse was defined as problematic use without compulsive use, tolerance, or withdrawal. The DSM-IV-TR (text revised, 2000) [7] revised the definition of substance abuse as meeting any one of four criteria that are substance-related and of dependence as meeting three or more of seven physiological or behavior criteria.

The DSM-5 (2013) [8] revisited the terminology and eliminated the categories of abuse and dependence. The transition was to avoid the one size fits all approach and the problem of "diagnostic orphans." The category of substance use disorders was established with different levels of severity (mild, moderate, and severe), determined by the number of diagnostic criteria met by an individual. Per the DSM-5, a diagnosis of substance use disorder is based on evidence of impaired control, social impairment, risky use, and pharmacological criteria. The DSM-5 marked an important recognition of understanding substance use disorders along a continuum of severity. Moving away from the categories of dependence and abuse was a major step to correct moralistic and pejorative language that is particularly linked to "abuse" and "abusers."

Where Is the Origin of Social Stigma and Pessimism?

Prior to being replaced by the disease model, the moral model of addiction—a view based on Christian morality—prevailed in the field until late 1970s and early 1980s. Per this model, the "addict" is a person who lacks the "moral fiber" to resist the urge. Similarly, the society labeled the "drunk" as a person lacking in moral character and unable to resist the temptation to give in to the "evil spirits" of alcohol.

The paper that I review next clarifies the differences between the compensatory self-control model and the more traditional disease approach to addictive disorders. Brickman and colleagues in the early 1980s wrote this fascinating attributional analysis of various models of helping and coping, and demonstrated that the determinants of etiology may be independent of determinants of change. *Models of Helping and Coping* [9] outlined a fourfold analysis of models of etiology and change that had significant relevance to addiction. Two questions were considered from an attributional perspective: (1) Is the individual (with addiction) considered to be personally responsible for the *development* (meaning etiology) of the addictive disorder (yes/no); and (2) Is the individual considered the person responsible for *changing* the problem (responsible for a solution) (yes/no)? The four models that emerge from this 2 × 2 contingency table are as following:

1. The disease/medical model assumes that the person is considered not responsible for the development of the addiction (victim of the disease) and that change is impossible unless the person seeks some kind of medical treatment (accepting help without being blamed for their weakness);
2. The moral model assumes that the person is to blame for becoming addicted (a sign of weak character due to a lack of willpower or moral fiber) and that the person is responsible for changing the addictive behavior;
3. The so-called enlightenment model holds that the person is to some extent responsible for initiating the addictive behavior but must work on giving up the notion of personal control in order to change the behavior (as in AA, where the person has to rely on a "higher power");
4. The compensatory model assumes that the person is not blamed for the problem but is still held responsible for solving it. In this model, the individual learns to "compensate" for a problem by assuming active responsibility and self-mastery in the change process; therefore, addiction is viewed as developing as a function of multiple biopsychosocial factors and not as a failure in personal will.

So, what do we learn from this paper? Each model provides a framework for understanding the problem and for formulating the change approach. Behavior change, such as abstinence, can be self-initiated—by the exercise of will power (moral model) and/or by acquiring compensatory coping skills (compensatory self-control model)—or by the outcome of professional treatment (medical model) or reliance on "higher power" as in AA (enlightenment model). Similarly, relapse (medical model term) can by conceptualized by each model as a return to use (a disease symptomatology, medical model), a sinful act (moral model), a result of losing connection with one's higher power (enlightenment model), or a mistake in compensatory coping (compensatory self-control model).

The traditional view of "alcoholism" using the American disease model implied that "alcoholics/addicts" are a separate class of people! In a commentary on the controlled drinking controversy, Marlatt [10] discussed the overlap between the disease model and the moral model as a major factor in the dispute:

> *"To some observers, the diagnosis of alcoholism carries the moral stigma of a new scarlet letter. Such critics argue that the contemporary disease model of addiction is little more than the old "moral model" (drinking as a sinful behavior) dressed up in sheep's clothing (or at least in a white coat). Despite the facts of the basic tenets of the disease model have yet to be verified scientifically (e.g., the physiological basis of the disease and its primary symptom, loss of control), and even though there is a lack of empirical support for the effectiveness of any particular form of alcoholism treatment (including inpatient programs geared towards abstinence), advocates of the disease model continue to insist that alcoholism is a unitary disorder, a progressive disease that can be temporarily arrested by total abstention. From this point of view, alcohol for the abstinent alcoholic symbolizes the forbidden fruit (a fermented apple) and a lapse from abstinence is tantamount to fall from grace in the eyes of God. Clearly one bite of the forbidden fruit is sufficient to be expelled from paradise. Anyone who suggests drinking is branded as an agent of the devil, tempting the naïve alcoholic back into the sin of drinking. If drinking is a sin, the only solution is salvation, a surrendering of personal control to a higher power."* (p. 1107)

Another greatly enlightening experience for me was reading the article written by Miller in 1986 [11] entitled *Haunted by the Zeitgeist: Reflections on Contrasting Treatment Goals and Concepts of Alcoholism in Europe and the United States*. This paper painted an insightful picture of where we, as a global society, were in terms of understanding "alcoholism" and the origin of the multiple assumptions and beliefs that it is a disease. I have revisited this article numerous times to capture a clear sense of how much the media and communities were so brainwashed by ideology instead of scientific evidence. Miller pointed out the importance of appreciating "the few empirical maps that we have and set off across the uncertain terrain in pursuit of mirages, even though the vision on the horizon be that of the great American dream of how alcoholism ought to be." Reviewing the disease or medical model of alcoholism, a few conclusions can be formulated for the "alcoholic or addict":

- "Alcoholics" have a disease that makes them constitutionally incapable of drinking in moderation.
- Their loss of control is permanent and irreversible.
- There is no known "cure" for the disease.
- "Alcoholism" is progressive, extending inexorably downwards to the depths of despair, and eventually death unless the condition is "arrested" by lifelong abstinence.
- "Alcoholics" use more primitive and immature defense mechanisms such as repression, denial, and turning hostility inward with a predisposing personality.
- Therefore, "alcoholics" are totally controlled by a powerful disease and out of touch with reality!

How do we challenge these perspectives using the scientific evidence?

- Substance use is a chosen *behavior* that responds to the same learning, social, environment, and cultural influences like other behaviors.
- There is no scientific evidence for the inevitable inherent loss of control. The reasons for the loss of control were assumed to be physiologically-related: a biomedical irreversible reaction to alcohol. A classic study by Marlatt and col-

leagues in 1973 [12], *Loss of Control Drinking in Alcoholics: An Experimental Analogue,* used a balanced placebo design in which some "alcoholics" were led to believe that they would be drinking alcohol, whereas others were told they would receive a non-alcoholic drink. Within each of these two groups, half received alcohol disguised in a mixer and half did not. Thus, there were "alcoholics" drinking alcohol and knowing it, others drinking alcohol without knowing it, others drinking a beverage that falsely believed to contain alcohol, and still others drinking only a mixer and knowing it. "Alcoholics" drank more of the beverage when they believed it to contain alcohol, whether or not it actually did. These results have been confirmed in multiple studies: drinking and experiencing craving appear to be triggered not by alcohol itself but by the *belief* that alcohol is present. Loss of control was triggered by "psychological" rather than "physiological" stimuli. More subsequent studies have shown that drinking behavior is substantially influenced by many psychological factors such as emotional states, social pressure, etc.

- There is no research evidence to support the belief that people with substance use disorders are different from others in using immature defense mechanisms. Research on different measures has shown the wide diversity of personality characteristics among people with addictions and their family members, who are as diverse as the general population [13]. There is absolutely no evidence of an addictive personality!
- The science of recovery has demonstrated that most people who recover from addictions do so on their own, without formal treatment. This "natural" change is not much different in terms of processes and form compared to change that occurs within treatment. The story of David Premack [14] serves as a good example. David quit smoking on a day in which he had gone to pick up his children at the city library. A thunderstorm greeted him as he arrived there. At the same time, a search of his pockets disclosed a familiar problem: he was out of cigarettes! Glancing back at the library on his way to buy cigarettes, he caught a glimpse of his children stepping out in the rain. Still, he continued around the corner, certain that he could find a parking space, rush in to the store, buy the cigarettes, and be back before the children got seriously wet. Identifying himself "as a father who could actually leave his kids in the rain while he ran after cigarettes" (p. 115) was a wake-up call that made him realize what is more important to him, and he quit smoking. It is worth noting, nevertheless, that effective interventions can facilitate and enhance the speed of the natural change process.
- The disease model justified and disseminated treatment approaches based on confrontation to break the immature defenses that were presumed to be linked to substance use disorders. Confrontation is delivered usually with the intent to evoke fear, shame, or humiliation. Two examples of therapeutic confrontation were described in a paper by White and Miller [15], *The Use of Confrontation in Addiction Treatment: History, Science, and Time for Change.* The first was from the Wall Street Journal (1983), describing a physician-led intervention with a corporate executive:

- When the executive tried to deny that he had a drinking problem, the medical director came down hard: "Shut up and listen," he said, "Alcoholics are liars, so we don't want to hear what you have to say." [16]
- The second example came from Chuck Dederich, the founder of Synanon, counseling a Mexican-American man with addiction in a therapeutic community, who balked at being ordered what to do: "Now, Buster, I am going to tell you what to do....that's the way we operate in Synanon: you see, you are getting a little emotional surgery. If you don't like the surgery, fine, go do what you have to do. Maybe we'll get you again after you get out of the penitentiary or after you get a drug overdose. 'Nobody tells me what to do!' Nobody in the world says that except dingbats like dope friends, alcoholics, and brush-faced covered El Gatos." ([17]; p. 122)
- Early in my training, some physicians stressed to me that confrontational interventions work very well with "addicts" and "alcoholics" to break their *denials*. I thought that it was the only way to deal with denial! Reflecting on my own experiences with patients, I realized that my perceptions of them being in *denial* occurred when I labeled them as "unmotivated" and when they disagreed with me about the treatment I recommended. Confronting them about not wanting to change made them angrier and more defensive, and they eventually refused to engage with me. A confrontational and authoritarian style clearly increases defensiveness and discord, not only in people with substance use disorders but in almost all human beings. In contrast, a listening and empathic style can substantially help reduce resistance and facilitate the process of change. At the time, there was a predominant belief that emotions and reactions generated by confrontation are therapeutic. In fact, expressed resistance in counseling sessions is predictive of a lack of subsequent behavior change [18]. The only way to avoid generating resistance and defensiveness is not to use confrontation! Reviewing four decades of treatment outcome research, there is *not* and has *never* been any scientific evidence for a therapeutic effect of confrontational interventions with substance use disorders. In fact, several studies reported harmful outcomes, including increased drop-out, more rapid relapse, and higher DWI (driving while intoxicated) recidivism.

- No evidence has been found to support the belief that the disease model reduces feelings of shame and stigma. The patient's belief in the disease model and lack of coping skills are two factors predictive of relapse to alcohol use.
- What seems clearer is that we have an integrated synthesis of behavioral, sociological, psychological, spiritual, and neurobiological factors that provides us with a more comprehensive empirical perspective on the nature of addictive disorders and how to treat them.

I can articulate with evidence and confidence that "alcoholics" and addicts" are not a separate species of people! Fundamental to my work in the field of addiction is to debunk the myths related to the perceptions that people with substance use disorders are a different category of people.

Reasons for Optimism and Hope: Key Issues in Treatment Effectiveness

Early data regarding the effectiveness of treatment were mostly focused on program evaluation studies and demonstrated that many individuals with substance use disorders did not seek treatment or access formal treatment; this unfortunately remains the case nowadays. Of the people who applied for treatment, many never followed through with their first appointment and many others dropped out very shortly after they initiated treatment. The subgroup of individuals who initiated and remained in treatment over longer periods of time had overall good outcomes, but relapse and recurrence of problems were significant. Throughout the years of my career, I have questioned how treatments are effective and how we define effectiveness. How do we define good outcome? How do we define relapse and treatment failure? And how do we describe "treatment"?

Reviewing two classic papers that I consider fundamental to understanding the effectiveness of treatments shed light on the evidence. The first paper is from 1986 by Miller and Hesler [19], *Inpatient Alcoholism Treatment: Who Benefits?* In the introduction, the authors reported that, in the early 1980s, there was an informal word of mouth "industry standard" of sorts in the U.S. in which it was common for programs to claim success rates of 80% or even higher! This article reviewed 26 controlled comparison studies that consistently showed *no* overall advantage for residential over nonresidential treatment settings, for longer over shorter inpatient programs, or for more intensive over less intensive interventions in treating alcohol use disorders. Intensive treatment may, however, be more beneficial for the more severely deteriorated and less socially stable individuals. This finding is extremely important as it indicates that the outcomes of inpatient programs were on average the same as those from less costly outpatient options. Another important finding from this review showed that the outcome of alcoholism treatment is more likely to be influenced by the *content* of interventions than by the settings in which they are delivered. We should strongly challenge the argument among healthcare practitioners that inpatient treatment is the gold standard for addiction treatment, because it simply is not science!

The second study, by Miller and colleagues [20], reviewed the outcomes for more than 8000 people treated for alcohol use disorders in seven multisite trials and showed that, during the year after treatment, 1.5% had died, 24% remained continuously abstinent for 12 months, and, among those who drank, alcohol use decreased by 87% and alcohol-related problems decreased by 60%. The substantial improvement in people who do not maintain "perfect" abstinence or moderation is overshadowed by a dichotomized approach ("successful" vs. "relapsed"). In fact, these outcomes have not changed substantially in 40 years. There is every reason to be optimistic and hopeful and to believe that addictions are treatable and their treatments are indeed effective!

The Effect of the Therapist in Addiction Treatment: Relationship Matters

One major research finding on the treatment of substance use disorders is that a significant determinant of patients' treatment outcome is the therapist with whom they work, regardless of the treatment approach. The reason is *empathy,* which is one of the strongest predictors of a therapist's effectiveness in treating substance use disorders. In one study, among nine therapists all delivering the same manual-guided behavioral therapy, patients' drinking outcomes were strongly predicted by the extent the therapist practiced accurate empathy (described in Chaps. 1 and 2) during treatment. Patients of the most empathic therapist (using Truax and Carkhuff's scale) showed a 100% improvement, whereas those of the least empathic therapist showed a 25% improvement rate [21]. Even 6 months, 1 year, and 2 years later, patients' drinking outcomes were strongly related to how empathic their therapist had been during treatment [22]. Another earlier study showed a strong relationship between patient relapse rates and the therapist's interpersonal skills using client-centered counseling. The more empathic and client-centered the therapist's style, the lower the relapse rate of the patient after counseling at 6, 12, 18, and 24 months [23]. On the other hand, some studies have demonstrated that certain therapists are outliers in terms of their patients having poor outcomes [24]. How we think about people within the context of therapy can make a significant difference, particularly about the belief in a patient's potential for change. In a well know classic study by Leake and King [25], the authors investigated whether counselors' expectations influenced the recovery of disadvantaged "alcoholics" of skid-row status. The authors informed therapists in three different treatment rehabilitation programs that they had conducted some psychological testing to identify patients with particularly high alcoholism recovery potential (HARP). The HARP patients were described as most likely to be successful in recovering from "alcoholism": They were more motivated, attended sessions on time, and worked harder in treatment. A year after discharge, the HARP patients who were assigned this optimistic prophecy at the initiation of treatment showed higher rates of abstinence, longer spans of abstinence, fewer slips, and more employment compared to patients of the control group. HARP and non-HARP patients did not differ from each other on prior treatment history or severity of alcoholism. In addition, the HARP patients identified as most likely to succeed had been chosen at random, and their therapists just believed they would do well. The therapist's expectations may significantly influence the adjustment and recovery of patients with alcohol use disorders. Believing in the patients' potential becomes a self-fulfilling prophecy. Another older study demonstrated that the voice tone of physicians who interviewed patients with alcoholism strongly predicted whether patients would complete the referral: the more anger and frustration in the physician's voice, the less likely it was the person would seek treatment [26].

Motivational Interviewing: My Path towards Clinical and Personal Transformation

"A word of informed consent: This approach is likely to change you" [27]. The approach of motivational interviewing (MI) originally evolved from Miller's practice with problem drinkers [28]. It is based on Rogers' client-centered counseling and conceptually is the opposite of confrontational interventions. The central aim of MI is to evoke from patients their intrinsic motivations for and commitment to change. It is complicated enough that one can put in a lifetime of work perfecting his or her use of the approach. It is not a set of techniques, and its style overrides its technical component. The research-based theory of its efficacy focuses on two components: a relational component and a technical component [29]. The relational component is based on the therapeutic alliance between practitioner and patient and is focused on accurate empathy. The relational component describes an underlying "spirit" of MI as a collaborative style: one that communicates acceptance, and respects and fully supports, patients' autonomy to choose and make decisions about their own lives and behaviors. It evokes from them their own insights, wisdom, and resources rather than trying to install things in them [30, 31]. This spirit affects the outcome. The technical piece is essentially the client-centered and non-authoritarian approach using the OARS skills (open-ended questions, affirmation, reflections, and summaries). Early in the development of MI, Rollnick and Miller particularly emphasized the essence of MI defined by the spirit that underlies the specific techniques:

> *"Impetus for change is drawn from the client's new intrinsic motives and goals, and it is the client who gives voice to reasons for change. Direct persuasion, coercion, and other saliently external controls are avoided. The therapeutic relationship has a partnership character, and the client's freedom of choice is emphasized."* ([30], p. 332)

A testimonial about the spirit of MI is expressed by John Eisenman, one of our therapists on the dual diagnosis unit:

> *"I have had the very humbling experience of working with MI for many years with people struggling with everything from acute trauma to self-discovery. I have witnessed the MI spirit reveal strength and understanding while delivering light and love to people who seemingly had explored every possible avenue of help. As therapists, we can usually see the desired outcome, yet we patiently wait for the individual to pick and travel their own path. The person then experiences the reality of self-efficacy and self-confidence. The MI spirit fills in the edges of the puzzle pieces they walk on, traveling the road to healing and growth. We are only trusted confidants of the true champions of the battle. People discover their personal truth. What a person chooses to do in their life belongs to them."*

When practicing MI, we aim to arrange the conversation so that people talk themselves into change. Thus, MI selectively elicits and reinforces motivational language such as change talk (desire, ability, reasons, and need: DARN) and commitment language. While the early psycholinguistic work of Amrhein [32] suggested only commitment language and DARN leading to commitment language predicted behavior change, further research has since shown that *any* change talk predicts behavior change and improves substance use outcomes [33, 34].

MI effectiveness is linked to the hope, deep respect, esteem, and faith in people and their resources, possibilities, and freedom to change. Additionally, motivational interviewing has been shown to be an effective strategy to reduce stigmatizing attitudes towards people with substance use disorders [35].

Reviewing the work of Dr. Miller in motivational factors in addictive behaviors and brief interventions including motivational interviewing demonstrated that relatively brief interventions can trigger significant change, and therapist empathy can be a strong predictor of patient change. In a classic paper published in 2000 titled *Rediscovering Fire: Small interventions, Large Effects* [36], Miller shared his struggles with understanding what triggers the phenomenon of change and debated ideas and theories. He discussed how parallel factors are often seen when change happens without formal treatment in a study of 55 individuals who described sudden and enduring transformations due to relatively brief experiences [37]. A commonality among them was that the experience involved qualities associated with *love*. A majority reported such experiences: "I felt completely loved"; "I felt at one with or connected to everything around me." Only a very small minority described feeling confused. These statements point to the experience of empathy and warmth, as it is related to the change process, even without formal treatment. Additionally, a shift in the value system was associated with the abrupt change. Prior to their experience, men reported that their five most important values were (in order): wealth, adventure, achievement, pleasure, and being respected. Post transformation, however, these values had changed considerably and had been replaced, respectively, by spirituality, personal peace, family, God's will, and honesty. Among women, priority shifts were also significant from pre-experience (family, independence, career, fitting in, and attractiveness) to post-experience (growth, self-esteem, spirituality, happiness, and generosity). The Scriptures speak of "renewed mind" as indicative of true change (e.g., Romans 12; Ephesians 1; Galatians 5).

The single English term *love* reflects four different words (concepts) from ancient Greek [38]. Three of them are not related to the therapy process (*philia*, *eros*, and *storge*). The fourth meaning, *agape*, was used in early Christianity to describe a selfless and sacred form of loving. Miller discussed the resemblance between agape—a quality of relating—and the critical conditions for change described by Carl Rogers [39, 40]. Based on the empirical data, highly effective therapists are believed to have in common many attributes such as empathy, selflessness, a positive view of the person, positive regard, and acceptance (one of the elements of the MI spirit). Acceptance describes the openness and curiosity about the patient's experiences and extends to the practitioner's own experiencing (genuineness in Rogerian's terms). The concept of agape also includes other attributes such as hope and patience. As discussed earlier in the chapter, the positive effects of faith and hopeful expectancy have been empirically well validated. A unique quality of the therapeutic relationship in the agape-driven spirit is the collaboration in the change process ("Come now, let us reason together": Isa. 1:18). "Dancing versus wrestling" was an earlier description of the partnership element of the MI spirit. Data from several studies have confirmed its impact, showing that the clinician and patient ratings of therapeutic "alliance" appear to be correlated with treatment outcome and retention [41]. Miller noted, "It is love and profound respect that are the music in motivational interviewing, without which the words are empty" (p. 13).

I am sharing with you this next personal experience because it was a turning point for me clinically and personally when I recognized and experienced the healing *love* of motivational interviewing. This is one of the most inspiring and memorable stories of my early clinical life that became the catalyst for the development of my professional calling. After more than 20 years of addiction practice, I still feel humbled by the mystery of the therapeutic impact of motivational interviewing.

My work with Jenny coincided with my introduction to practicing motivational interviewing. Given that, our work was often uneven as I found my footing with this new "discovery." In some sessions, I felt awkward, inauthentic, or preoccupied with the details of MI. Other times, I felt relaxed and as though the approach facilitated our work and relationship in a powerful way. Jenny had a bright and compelling personality, and was pleasant to work with when she was feeling balanced and euthymic. Nevertheless, our work together certainly had some difficult patches. My use of the MI spirit and strategies in these rough spots was helpful in moving our work along with little conflict, and may have helped to provide a new experience I think Jenny carried with her as she moved on. Jenny fixated on medication interventions as the major solution to her struggles at the beginning of our treatment. Using MI to navigate the clinical interaction, I let Jenny become my "best teacher." I offered, with her permission, that changing her substance use behavior and working to process her traumatic experiences linked to her addiction would potentially help her live a life consistent with her expectation of herself. At first, she was angry at this suggestion. Through accurate empathy (via reflective listening), demonstration of respect of her autonomy, and rolling with her objections, she dramatically changed her mind and accepted my perspective. In a major instance in our work, as she was suffering from mild withdrawal symptoms, she sat with me and made the case for needing more medication. She became angry with me at times, criticized me, and accused me of withholding something she needed just to inflict her with pain. I reflected her anger and calmly told her that I could see her suffering and shared that I did not see any clinical indication to change the medication regimen. I told her that I would continue to work with her even if she disagreed with my decision. I could see her working to regulate her anger. The following day, she apologized for having been angry with me.

On her discharge day, she reiterated this point, saying that it was important that I had remained calm, nonjudgmental, compassionate, and respectful when she was upset with me. In the past, others had always responded in kind, leading to escalated hostility and subsequently to her shutting down.

We were discussing her previously held belief that her drug use did not affect her son when I realized, as I was reflecting, that there had been a change in her thinking. I had previously worked hard to continue listening and reflecting what she would say as I felt heat in my chest and a pressure to tell her how much her use affected her son. Then, I embraced my faith in MI!

My experience with Jenny strengthened my belief that change was within her own reach and guided by the MI spirit and strategies. All I had to do was to activate her motivation, wisdom, and value system. I learned accurate empathy from working with her and experienced its impact on her recovery. I knew that I was likely to worry about how she was doing with her recovery. I knew I would also worry about that son of hers whom I have never met.

The following clinical reflection shared by a former medical student (Annie Lu) during her psychiatry rotation on the dual diagnosis unit with me offers perspectives on the ambiguities and struggles of patients labeled as "difficult." She not only explores the ways in which motivational interviewing addresses the patient's problems, but also illuminates its impact on her and how we can conceptualize the unpredictable ways in which change occurs:

> "When I first interviewed Roy, we sat alone in the treatment room, and I admit I was frightened of him. He had come from out of town with a friend to "hit all the hospitals in town" for opioid pain medications, and presented to the emergency room requesting detoxification after his friend abandoned him and left him stranded, broke, and in a state of withdrawal. When I first engaged him on the inpatient unit, he seemed calm, sitting hunched over and staring at the ground, but his words and monotonous tone of voice suggested a seething anger and misery that I worried could turn explosive if I said the wrong thing. As I got to know Roy, it became apparent that his potential for violence was the least difficult challenge I would face in working with him. As our team began working with him, we found no shortage of reasons to feel thoroughly irritated by him. In my most unforgiving moments, I thought Roy to be manipulative, entitled, and demanding. He victimized himself instead of taking responsibility for his actions. Despite recognizing the devastating state of his current life, he exhibited a persistent narcissism, often boasting about his high IQ, outstanding altruism, and extensive knowledge of 12-step programs. On top of this, he continually sought medications despite having completed detoxification, and was deceitful about previous treatment courses.
>
> William R. Miller and Stephen Rollnick make an analogy between working with an ambivalent patient towards change and following a lighthouse signal (the patient's desire to change) through the noise of a storm (patient's desire to keep using). Working with Roy could not have been a better opportunity to put this into practice. In his case, the noise obscuring his recovery was not only his desire to keep using, but also his borderline and narcissistic traits. These traits not only made it difficult for him to recognize his responsibility for the decisions he made, but also made it difficult for our team to empathize with his struggles.
>
> After each session with Roy in our treatment team, we debriefed and often found ourselves irritated and ranting disgustedly about the personality traits we had found repelling. At the same time, I learned that it was possible to focus on the lighthouse through the storm, to detach myself from these negative impressions and focus on his treatment with a more dispassionate approach. During our team discussions, we discussed hypotheses for what might be driving Roy's attitudes and behaviors. We considered his addiction from the perspective of his inability to cope with feelings of loss, anger, shame, and anxiety in his life, leading him to seek escape and relief in the medications he abused. We considered his disproportionate anger at staff and patients from the perspective of him externalizing his fears in the face of a possible serious medical issue that we were working up during his admission. We considered his demanding manner and lack of negotiation skills from the perspective of him going through life as a large intimidating man, for whom these tactics have often been successful in getting him what he wants. When Roy was open to hearing our observations and hypotheses, we shared these ideas with him. Although his narcissism and sense of entitlement remained strong and as repelling to me as ever, I saw him slowly begin to focus more on the working on himself. By the end of his inpatient stay, he was learning to acknowledge and reflect on some of his own shortcomings, and finally identify a few of his own goals for his recovery. These were significant achievements for him.

Working with Roy, whose personality tends to push away the people who try to help him, I realized that it is often the patients who are most difficult to empathize with who stand to benefit the most from our patience, positive regard, and understanding. Empathizing with Roy required recognizing that "difficult" patients do not emerge from a vacuum. Their thoughts, feelings, behaviors, and personality can be explored in terms of the life experiences and emotional processes that shaped them, and, once these histories are uncovered, they become opportunities for change and growth. Putting the lighthouse analogy into practice was one of the most challenging aspects of working with Roy, who taught me that without a deliberate and disciplined focus on a patient's beacon of opportunity for change, one is almost surely fated to get lost in the storm."

Relapse Prevention

The revolutionary work of Marlatt and his colleagues in the early 1970s [12] that led to the introduction of relapse prevention theory and model (RP) in the early 1980s challenged the prevailing disease model of addictions and provided a new paradigm for our understanding of the determinants of relapse. It formulated stronger, more hopeful evidence that loss of control as well as relapse (tenets of the disease model) need not be inevitable. Since loss of control does not have to be a binding outcome of taking a drink, it might be possible to prevent future drinking behaviors by modifying many malleable individual variables such as expectancies and environmental factors. This notion has major clinical implications and has evolved into bettering the distinction between a "lapse" (initial breaking of abstinence) and a "relapse" (going back to the unhealthy behavior following a lapse). These findings have challenged the need for total abstinence and introduced the development of harm reduction approaches incorporating relapse prevention strategies [42, 43]. Subsequent clinical observations and research findings identified situational and emotional factors that immediately precede relapse [44]. The resultant taxonomy of high-risk situations contributing to relapse consisted of two domains:

- The first domain, *Intrapersonal Determinants,* includes situations such as coping with negative emotional states; coping with physical discomfort; reinforcing positive emotional states; challenging one's willpower using a substance; and giving in to urges and cravings to use substances;
- The second domain, *Interpersonal Determinants,* includes situations such as coping with interpersonal conflicts; social pressure to use; and strengthening positive emotional states in social encounters and relationships.

If these high-risk situations could be identified early in the process and addressed through effective coping, the probability of lapse and relapse could be reduced. This led to the conceptualization of RP therapy. Additional research evaluating the efficacy of skills training interventions in patients with substance use disorders provided more empirical support for Marlatt RP theory and RP therapy. The classic 1985 publication of the book *Relapse Prevention: Maintenance Strategies in the*

Treatment of Addictive Behaviors [44] discussed comprehensively the RP theoretical model and its clinical applications across a spectrum of addictive behaviors. Reasons for optimism and hope were related to the basic assumptions of the RP model that patients with substance use disorders could potentially prevent relapse, improve treatment outcome, and reduce the negative consequences of addictive behaviors. The adoption and clinical application of the RP model evolved through the dissemination process that was initiated by Dennis Daley, which was patient-focused and treatment-directed [45–49]. Dennis Daley became very much involved in RP through developing clinical programs and interventions disseminating Marlatt's work via writings, videos, and workbooks. The first workbook for patients, *Relapse Prevention Workbook: For Recovering Alcohol and Drug Dependent Persons*, was focused on helping patients become better informed and skillful in coping with relapse-related issues [46]. This workbook has been edited and updated several times. Concomitantly, Dennis Daley developed a therapist manual discussing the RP model and interventions conceptualized as a curriculum for a 12-session group-based RP intervention that was used with the interactive workbook for patients [46]. This intervention was adapted to different treatment settings for individuals with substance use disorders [50]. Donovan and Witkiewitz [51] described the collaboration between Alan Marlatt and Dennis Daley as "a tremendous combination and blending of a brilliant theoretician and a skilled practitioner and program implementer." Research on RP kept evolving over the course of years, and, to date, the efficacy and effectiveness of RP and treatments that incorporate elements of RP have been well established. Miller and Wilbourne [52] reviewed treatments that were ranked among the top ten treatments for alcohol use disorders (Mesa Grande) based on effect sizes and methodological quality, including brief interventions, social skills training, behavioral marital therapy, and self-monitoring. These approaches incorporated aspects of RP and were largely based on the cognitive-behavioral model of relapse. McCrady [53] pointed out that "Marlatt's RP model dramatically changed the way the treatment community conceptualized relapse" (p. 1015).

Pharmacological Treatments

The role of pharmacotherapy in the treatment of substance use disorders depends considerably on the substance of abuse. Medications can play a major role in the initial attainment of abstinence (pharmacologically-assisted detoxification) and in prevention of relapse. It is wrong to believe that letting patients suffer during the withdrawal process make them more motivated for recovery. Medication-assisted treatments are fundamental to the treatment of opioid use disorder, in combination with behavioral interventions that can enhance adherence and retention in treatment. Similarly, in the same context, an effective pharmacological approach may help a patient engage better in treatment, thereby allowing the patient to utilize the skills learned from the behavioral interventions. Effective pharmacotherapy for addictions can play an important role in primary health care settings. Healthcare practitioners in these settings should be able to screen, evaluate, do a brief intervention, prescribe, and monitor the response to treatment [54]. In fact, people with substance use disorders can benefit from pharmacotherapy delivered within primary care settings [54]. The evidence demonstrates that addiction treatment can be initiated or even done in non-specialized medical settings. This is particularly important since many people with substance use disorders do not seek and do not receive treatment within an addiction specialty program. Debunking myths related to ideology and stigma about pharmacotherapy for addictive disorders is necessary to remove barriers to prescribing in medical settings. Clearly, the responsible and clinically appropriate prescribing patterns in the treatment of substance use disorders remains a major challenge in the addiction treatment field.

Seven Robust Scientific Findings Informing Clinical Practices

1. There is significant evidence indicating *no* connection between therapeutic effectiveness and one's own history of addiction. Personal recovery status does not have an added value to one's therapeutic work, even when delivering 12-step-based treatment [24]. It neither increases nor decreases one's success in treating substance use disorders. As discussed earlier, therapeutic effectiveness is correlated with therapeutic empathy and other attributes.
2. What we need in order to create an effective substance use treatment system is an integration of a comprehensive, interdisciplinary, evidence-based, collaborative, and holistic care approach.
3. Unlike other areas of healthcare, treatment of substance use disorders may be the only area of medical care in which there is a specialty care without any primary care [55]. Patients with substance use disorder are very rarely referred to specialty care from a primary care physician. A wealth of evidence has accumulated throughout the years indicating the benefits of brief physician advice, brief motivational interventions and/or screening, brief intervention, and referral to treatment (SBIRT) in primary and specialty medical care settings for reducing alcohol and substance use, at least in the short term [56, 57]. Furthermore, brief interventions are associated with improvements in emotional problems, higher rates of employment, and reduction in mortality rate [56, 58]. It is time to integrate brief interventions in all healthcare settings including dentistry, pharmacy, employee assistance programs, and even social services.
4. The longer patients have to wait to receive treatment services, the less likely it is that they will follow through and engage [59]. When patients make the decision to seek treatment, they take the risk of being stigmatized. Having to wait for treatment may constitute a loss of a "teachable moment." It is time to end waiting lists!
5. Identification of substance use disorders, treatment linkage, engagement in treatment services, and therapeutic outcome are hindered by:

(a) Social stigma and pessimism (among the public, healthcare practitioners, and even patients themselves) about the possibility of change [60, 61];
(b) Criminalization of people who use substances; obstacles to accessing services, including transportation issues (the treatment center being a long distance from the patient's home, for example), and lack of insurance benefits;
(c) Societal perspectives and approaches to substance use disorders as moral failings rather than treatable chronic medical illnesses;
(d) Public perceptions influenced by ideas such as nothing can be done until the person "hits bottom" and is ready to change. That "culture of addiction" promotes the wrong treatment approach. In fact, positive reinforcement and brief motivational interventions have been demonstrated to mobilize the process of change in "unmotivated" individuals. We cannot afford to wait for the person to be totally highjacked by the addiction to become ready. We need to intervene as early as possible so we can enhance motivation for change.

6. Polydrug use is the expectation not the exception. Additionally, individuals who seek treatment for either a psychiatric problem or a substance use disorder are more likely to have a co-occurring disorder than individuals with a disorder who do not seek treatment, a phenomenon known as "Berkson's fallacy." Comorbidity of substance use and psychiatric disorders is a dominant clinical presentation in most treatment settings. Traditionally segregated treatments providing separate psychiatric and substance use treatments such as parallel or sequential treatment approaches have proved to be ineffective. In contrast to these approaches, integrated treatment models addressing co-occurring substance use and psychiatric disorders have strong empirical evidence, particularly for patients with severe psychiatric disorders.
7. Retention is a consistent predictor of substance use treatment outcome. Patients with drug use disorders with longer episodes of residential or outpatient care experience better substance use and crime-related outcomes than do patients with shorter episodes [62, 63]. The finding that the duration of treatment for substance use disorders is more closely related to better outcome than the amount or intensity of treatment is congruent with the process of recovery. NIDA Principles of Drug Treatment made it clear that any treatment less than 90 days of care—at whatever levels—is of questionable value [64].

References

1. American Psychiatric Association. Diagnostic and statistical manual of mental disorders. Washington, DC: American Psychiatric Association; 1952.
2. American Psychiatric Association. Diagnostic and statistical manual of mental disorders. Washington, DC: American Psychiatric Association; 1968.
3. Jellinek EM. The disease concept of alcoholism. Highland Park, NJ: Hillhouse Press; 1960.

4. American Psychiatric Association. Diagnostic and statistical manual of mental disorders. Washington, DC: American Psychiatric Association; 1980.
5. American Psychiatric Association. Diagnostic and statistical manual of mental disorders. Washington, DC: American Psychiatric Association; 1987.
6. American Psychiatric Association. Diagnostic and statistical manual of mental disorders. Washington, DC: American Psychiatric Association; 1994.
7. American Psychiatric Association. Diagnostic and statistical manual of mental disorders. Washington, DC: American Psychiatric Association; 2000.
8. American Psychiatric Association. Diagnostic and statistical manual of mental disorders. Washington, DC: American Psychiatric Association; 2013.
9. Brickman P, Rabinowitz VC, Karuza J, Coates D, Cohn E, Kidder L. Models of helping and coping. Am Psychol. 1982;37(4):368–84.
10. Marlatt GA. The controlled-drinking controversy: a commentary. Am Psychol. 1983;38(10):1097–110.
11. Miller WR. Haunted by the zeitgeist: reflections on contrasting treatment goals and concepts of alcoholism in Europe and the United States. Ann N Y Acad Sci. 1986;472(1):110–29.
12. Marlatt GA, Demming B, Reid JB. Loss of control drinking in alcoholics: an experimental analogue. J Abnorm Psychol. 1973;81(3):233.
13. Donovan DM, Hague WH, O'Leary MR. Perceptual differentiation and defense mechanisms in alcoholics. J Clin Psychol. 1975;31(2):356–9.
14. Premack D. Mechanisms of self-control. In: Learning mechanisms in smoking. Chicago: Aldine; 1970. p. 107–23.
15. White WL, Miller WR. The use of confrontation in addiction treatment: history, science and time for change. Counselor. 2007;8(4):12–30.
16. Greenberger RS. Sobering method: firms are confronting alcoholic executives with threat of firing. Wall St J. 1983;1:26.
17. Yablonsky L. Synanon: the tunnel back. Baltimore: Penguin Books; 1965.
18. Miller WR, Hedrick KE, Taylor CA. Addictive behaviors and life problems before and after behavioral treatment of problem drinkers. Addict Behav. 1983;8(4):403–12.
19. Miller WR, Hester RK. Inpatient alcoholism treatment: who benefits? Am Psychol. 1986;41:794–805.
20. Miller WR, Walters ST, Bennett ME. How effective is alcoholism treatment in the United States? J Stud Alcohol. 2001;62:211–20.
21. Miller WR, Taylor CA, West JC. Focused versus broad spectrum behavior therapy for problem drinkers. J Consult Clin Psychol. 1980;48(5):590–601.
22. Miller WR, Baca LM. Two-year follow-up of bibliotherapy and therapist-directed controlled drinking training for problem drinkers. Behav Ther. 1983;14:441–8.
23. Valle SK. Interpersonal functioning of alcoholism counselors and treatment outcome. J Stud Alcohol. 1981;42(9):783–90.
24. Project Match Research Group. Therapist effects in three treatments for alcohol problems. Psychother Res. 1998;8:455–74.
25. Leake GJ, King AS. Effect of counselor's expectations on alcoholic recovery. Alcohol Health Res World. 1977;11(3):16–22.
26. Milmoe S, Rosenthal R, Blane HT, Chafetz ME, Wolf I. The doctor's voice: post-editor of successful referral of alcoholic patients. J Abnorm Psychol. 1967;72(1):78.
27. Miller WR, Rollnick S. Motivational interviewing: preparing people to change addictive behavior. New York: Guilford Publications; 1991.
28. Miller WR. Motivational interviewing with problem drinkers. Behav Psychother. 1983;11:147–72.
29. Miller WR, Rose GS. Towards a theory of motivational interviewing. Am Psychol. 2009;64(6):527–37.

30. Rollnick S, Miller WR. What is motivational interviewing? Behav Cogn Psychother. 1995;23(4):325–34.
31. Miller WR, Rollnick S. Motivational interviewing: helping people change. New York: Guilford Press; 2013.
32. Amrhein PC, Miller WR, Yahne CE, Palmer M, Fulcher L. Client commitment language during motivational interviewing predicts drug use outcomes. J Consult Clin Psychol. 2003;31:756–84.
33. Moyers TB, Martin T, Houck JM, Christopher PJ, Tonigan JS. From in-session behaviors to drinking outcomes: a causal chain for motivational interviewing. J Consult Clin Psychol. 2009;77(6):1113–24.
34. Magill M, Gaume J, Apocada TR, Wathers J, et al. The technical hypothesis of motivational interviewing: a meta-analysis of MI's key causal model. J Consult Clin Psychol. 2014;82(6):973–83.
35. Livingston JD, Milne T, Fang ML, Amari E. The effectiveness of interventions for reducing stigma related to substance use disorders: a systematic review. Addiction. 2012;107(1):39–50.
36. Miller WR. Rediscovering fire: small interventions, large effects. Psychol Addict Behav. 2000;14(1):6–18.
37. Miller WR, C'de BJ. Quantum change: when epiphanies and sudden insight transform ordinary lives. New York: Guilford Press; 2001.
38. Lewis C. The four loves: the much beloved exploration of the nature of love. New York: Harcourt; 1960.
39. Rogers CR. Client-centered therapy. Washington, DC: American Psychological Association; 1966.
40. Rogers CR. A way of being. New York: Houghton Mifflin Harcourt; 1995.
41. Luborsky L, Auerbach A. The therapeutic relationship in psychodynamic psychotherapy: the research evidence and its meaning for practice. Psychiatry Update: The American psychiatric association annual review, 1985.
42. Marlatt GA, Witkiewitz K. Harm reduction approaches to alcohol use: health promotion, prevention, and treatment. Addict Behav. 2002;27(6):867–86.
43. Larimer ME, Marlatt GA. Applications of relapse prevention with moderation goals. J Psychoactive Drugs. 1990;22(2):189–95.
44. Marlatt GA, Gordon JR. Relapse prevention: maintenance strategies in the treatment of addictive behaviors. New York: Guilford Press; 1985.
45. Cummings C, Gordon JR, Marlatt GA. Relapse: Strategies of prevention and prediction. In W. R. Miller (Ed.), The addictive behaviors. Oxford, England; Pergamon Press; 1980. p. 291–321.
46. Daley DC. Relapse prevention workbook. Holmes Beach, FL: Learning Publications Inc; 1986.
47. Daley DC. Relapse prevention: treatment alternatives and counseling aids. Blaze Ridge Summit, PA: TAB Books; 1989.
48. Daley DC, Marlatt GA. Relapse prevention: cognitive and behavioral interventions. In: Lowinson JH, editor. Substance abuse: a comprehensive textbook. Baltimore: Williams and Wilkins; 1992. p. 533–42.
49. Daley DC, Marlatt GA. Relapse prevention. In: Lowinson JH, editor. Substance abuse: a comprehensive textbook. Baltimore: Williams and Wilkins; 1997. p. 458–67.
50. Daley DC, Douaihy A. Relapse prevention counseling strategies: strategies to aid recovery from addiction and reduce relapse risk. Murrysville, PA: Daley Publication; 2011.
51. Donovan D, Witkiewitz W. Relapse prevention: from radical idea to common practice. Addict Res Theory. 2012;20(3):204–17.
52. Miller WR, Wilbourne PL. Mesa Grande: a methodological analysis of clinical trials of treatments for alcohol use disorders. Addiction. 2002;97(3):265–77.
53. McCrady B. In remembrance: G. Alan Marlatt. Alcohol Clin Exp Res. 2011;35(6):1015–6.
54. Saitz R. Unhealthy alcohol use. N Engl J Med. 2005;352(6):596–607.

55. McLellan TM. What we need is a system: creating a responsive and effective substance abuse treatment system. In: Miller WR, Carroll KM, editors. Rethinking substance abuse: what the science shows and we should do about it. New York: Guilford Press; 2006. p. 286.
56. Madras B, Campton W, Avula D, et al. Screening, brief intervention, and referral to treatment (SBIRT) for illicit drug and alcohol use at multiple healthcare sites. Camparison at intake and 6 months later. Drug Alcohol Depend. 2009;99:280–95.
57. D'Onofrio G, Degutis L. Integrating project ASSERT: a screening, intervention, and referral to treatment for unhealthy alcohol and drug use into an urban emergency department. Acad Emerg Med. 2010;17:903–11.
58. Cuijpers P, Riper H, Lemmers L. The effects on mortality of brief intervention fro problem drinking: a meta-analysis. Addiction. 2004;99:839–54.
59. Carroll KM. Improving compliance with alcoholism treatment (Project MATCH, Monographs series, vol 6). Rockville, MD: NIAAA. 1997.
60. Moyers TB, Miller WR. Therapists' conceptualizations of alcoholism: measurement and implications for treatment decisions. Psychol Addict Behav. 1993;7(4):238.
61. Schomerus G, Corrigan PW, Klauer T, Kuwert P, Freyberger HJ, Lucht M. Self-stigma in alcohol dependence: consequences for drinking-refusal self-efficacy. Drug Alcohol Depend. 2011;114(1):12–7.
62. Crits-Christoph P, Siqueland L. Psychosocial treatment for drug abuse: selected review and recommendations for national health care. Arch Gen Psychiatry. 1996;53(8):749–56.
63. Prendergast ML, Podus D, Chang E. Program factors and treatment outcomes in drug dependence treatment: an examination using meta-analysis. Subst Use Misuse. 2000;35(12–14):1931–65.
64. Principles of Drug Addiction Treatment: A research-based guide (third edition). National Institute on Drug Abuse, 2012. https://www.drugabuse.gov/publications/principles-addiction-treatment-research-based-guide-third-edition. Accessed 15 Jan 2018.

Chapter 5
Working with Family and Significant Others

> *"There is no doubt that it is around the family and the home that all the greatest values, the most dominating virtues of human society, are created, strengthened, and maintained."*
> —Winston Churchill

> *"The sun looks down on nothing half so good as a household laughing together over a meal."*
> —C. S. Lewis, 1949 [1]

Introduction

Treatment of substance use disorders has mostly focused on the "identified" patient with the addiction. Nevertheless, a key treatment principle remains to mobilize the family as a crucial resource whenever possible. Involvement of family members and concerned significant others (CSOs) has been sometimes thought to add an unpredictable level of complexity to what has otherwise been seen in some ways a journey that belongs to the patient alone. Clinical experience has borne out that engaging families as resources complicates the dynamics of treatment primarily when healthcare practitioners themselves are not well trained in working with couples, families, and CSOs. As Churchill intimates, "the individual is known and knows herself in the context of some kind of family." One might add that it is the family that is the stuff of larger workings (that evolve over time): social and community networks of CSOs, friends, coworkers, and neighbors. To conceive of an individual's struggles with addiction (and its treatment!) through the lens of relationships with loved ones is to already consider how to fortify a treatment plan with supports for which there is no substitute.

Certain ethnic groups harbor within them some powerful social and community resources which may be uniquely harnessed for therapeutic ends. One example of a group that influences the dynamics of family and extended kin networks is the African American culture, which has in it the church community as an important component of the social network. Similarly, for Native Americans, the extended kin network is regarded as central to everyday activities and ceremonies. People with alcohol and drug use disorders are considerably influenced by their social networks. Family relationships can either contribute to the maintenance of substance use problems or help an individual who uses substances to identify the problem and seek help. There are also two major scientifically-driven reasons for involving and working with families and CSOs: first, doing so can significantly enhance positive outcomes which increase the individual's chances of recovery; and secondly, adult family members and children can be negatively affected by the addiction and need support and help themselves [2–4].

Myths About Families and Addiction

The bidirectional relationship between substance use behavior and one's interpersonal relationships has been well established. Research has shown that a disproportionate number of relationships end after addiction treatment for multiple reasons including a cascade of conflict and relationship distress [5]. Additionally, we know that an interpersonal conflict with a CSO is the main determinant of people resuming substance use [6, 7]. Therefore, in recovery work, addressing relationship issues is as important as addressing the individual's substance use.

Various hypotheses have been discussed over the years about the link between addiction and the family. The first one is the *disturbed spouse hypothesis*. It posits that these spouses have deep-seated personality problems that stem from disturbances in childhood. It also implies that the spouse uses "enabling" behaviors (a term associated with family behaviors that promote the continuation of substance use) to sabotage the partner's attempts to quit drinking. Furthermore, it implies that if the partner were to achieve sobriety, the spouse would decompensate [8]. The second one is the *disturbed family hypothesis*. It is closely related to family systems theory which postulates that the pathology is attributed to the dysfunctional patterns of family interaction. This theory identifies each family member with a pathological role that maintains the equilibrium of the disturbed family system. Per this hypothesis, the family would be expected to hinder recovery, if not even sabotage it. Within these family dynamics, enabling behaviors would help restore the equilibrium and prevent deterioration of the family [9]. The third one is the *codependence hypothesis* [10, 11]. Per this hypothesis, addiction is a "family disease" whereby the person with the addiction and the "family members are afflicted with complementary and interlocking illnesses" [12]. The "disease of codependence or codependency" refers to the personality pathology of family members and is perceived to be related to the "addictive personality." The manifestations of codependence include emotional pain, high propensity for inappropriate behavior, dishonesty, and denial of the illness and the need for help [13]. The gridlock of pathology in this hypothesis implies that family members need separate treatment to address their codependent tendencies. Problematically, these three hypotheses posit that the spouse or the whole family have some sort of pathology independent of the family member with the addiction.

Scientific evidence demonstrates *no support* whatsoever for any of these hypotheses [14]. The very terms and concepts themselves cloud our conception of family and how to use its strengths to help the patient: the American Psychiatric Association has rejected the very term "codependence" as a diagnostic category because of lack of empirical evidence. Furthermore, a study that looked at the broader impact of behavioral self-control training intervention focusing on the reduction of alcohol consumption showed that most other life problems improved at all follow-up points, from 3 months to 2 years [15]. So we know that rallying an individual's family resources is not a liability.

Much of the early literature [16, 17] regarding the process of family adjustment and coping with a loved one with an addiction discussed the stages that address recognition of disorder development, discontinuation of use, treatment and early recovery, and ongoing recovery [18]. One key concept within the first stage is the stigmatizing behaviors of what is known as *enabling*. Understanding this concept is essential to understanding the development of the disorder process. To "enable" means to facilitate or aid a process. However, in the addiction process, enabling results in negative outcomes, in part by protecting the addicted individual from the negative consequences of the addictive behaviors which can present helpful learning opportunities within the addiction experience. In short, enabling interferes with the natural personal and societal consequences of the addiction, which inadvertently contributes to its continued progression [18]. Examples of enabling behaviors include buying alcohol or drugs for the individual to use or giving money to the individual to use for the same purpose. Paying fines related to use and covering up the serious consequences of use are other examples. One evidence-based approach to build awareness of the process of enabling is the CRAFT method (Community Reinforcement and Family Training). It aims to work with CSOs to provide positive reinforcement for non-substance using behaviors and engage ambivalent loved ones in addiction treatment [19, 20]. This framework is elaborated in more detail later in this chapter.

Impact of Substance Use Disorders on Family and Children

Patients with substance use disorders cannot be understood and treated effectively without consideration of the impact of the addiction on the family [18]. The evidence is strong for the negative effects of substance use on the family, particularly on spouses, parents, and children [3, 21]. Substance use impacts a wide range of family systems and processes, including family rituals, roles, family activities, communication skills, family social life, and finances. Families in which a parent has a substance use disorder often have a toxic environment characterized by fear, loss, grief, secrecy, conflict, violence, and role reversal. Parents' substance use is associated with more childhood stressors such as parental neglect, disruption of family rituals and activities, and physical and sexual abuse. Violence and child abuse are prevalent in families with a member with addiction, and these issues should be addressed preventively and in treatment. The consequences of these and other behaviors contribute to the development of high levels of physical and emotional distress in family members. In addition, we know from significant research evidence that children of parents with drug and alcohol problems are more likely to have poor school performance, depression, and delinquency [22, 23]. Furthermore, they are more likely to develop problems with substances themselves, with an early onset of use [24]. On the other hand, there is strong evidence that not all children are affected negatively, either as children or adults [25]. Some of these children are resilient and do not develop psychological disturbances. Furthermore, co-occurring psychiatric disorders can negatively affect the family unit, individual family members, CSOs, and children. In conclusion, family members need support and help, both for themselves and in relation to coping with their relationship with their loved one with substance use or co-occurring psychiatric disorders.

Scott was a patient I worked with during his inpatient treatment on the dual diagnosis unit. He was admitted after he took a serious overdose on psychotropics and heroin. Tough and guarded, he was articulate and widely seen as engaging and affable by the staff on the unit. He had returned for admission after being "administratively discharged" 2 months earlier due to possession of cannabis on the unit. When I engaged him in the first session, he shared that he had been thinking a lot about his life and that he had a wake-up call. He thought that maybe he did not want to die. He shared openly with us his belief that he was meant to be here for a reason while simultaneously discussing his difficulty in asking for our help, especially regarding his depression and addiction. His fear of discussing these emotional and behavioral vulnerabilities stemmed from "my father and stepfather would tell me to man up, that I am weak, and that psychiatrists would fool me into using some other drug." However, he remembered how, before he started using substances, he used to feel comfortable sharing with his mother about his struggles and that this sharing made him feel more secure. At the time of his admission, he reported that he would keep his feelings bottled up inside until he felt overwhelmed, and he would choose to snort heroin because it "cleared his mind," "made him calm," and gave him "problem-solving abilities." In our sessions, he identified these difficulties in regulating his own mental and emotional processes without drugs as a serious problem. The last time he got high to solve a problem was related to mounting financial pressure which he decided to deal with by choosing to rob a bank. After devastating personal experiences related to the consequences of his use, he was fed up with his life and decided to try to end his life. This time, though, he insisted that he was in a different place than the time he was in treatment only 2 months ago.

During the week that I worked with him, he slowly allowed me into his life. He told me about a life of repeated traumatic experiences while living in a poor neighborhood where he witnessed deaths and violence, and experienced physical abuse. He shared that he was "hardened" and became tougher, and started spending more time on the streets of a nearby drug-infested neighborhood, running with gang members. He ended up moving out of his house into that neighborhood and joining the gang because he felt more of a "sense of belonging" within the atmosphere of violence and danger in which people rarely used words to resolve conflicts. These experiences drove him to heroin use, which turned him into the "impulsive and selfish person" that he had come to know and despise. His gang lifestyle and heroin use were intertwined. As a higher-ranking gang member, he was close to heroin dealers and they would give him free drugs. He also felt pressure to use among some of his associates to deal with his inhibitions about acting unlawfully when he felt he had to prove himself within the gang he felt he belonged to. If he was in that environment, he had an exciting life that he could let go of no more easily than the heroin that he depended on to stimulate his mind. He could hit the streets, make money, and score drugs, all of which for him led to intense, irreproducible highs. At the same time, he longed for a more settled life with his wife and children, who "mean the world to me." Ultimately, he decided that his family was the reason he wanted to and needed to change.

His family came to visit him several times during his treatment. He asked me to join him for an impromptu family session while his mother, wife, and cousin were visiting. First, his mother shared how she was wary about his stated desire to stop using; she had seen him try many times and felt the sting of his broken promises just as often. Burned and weary, she had almost given up hope on him. In these sessions, he slowly shared his traumatic experiences that left him with deep guilt and shame and drove him to use heroin. His wife wept while he spoke, thinking she might finally be able to reconnect with the "good" person she always thought that he was deep down inside. He shared more about the person whom he believed he was meant to be and the values that defined him: kindness, compassion, dutifulness, and devotedness to his family.

He spoke movingly about wanting to be a good father to his children, unlike both of his own fathers. He talked about how one father was also addicted to drugs, and how his own dad was in and out of jail as well as in and out of his life. He wanted to make sure that he could be there for his children and set them on the right path so they would not follow in his footsteps and those of his father before him. One of the most striking events that changed his attitude about life was when his son put a bandana on his head like a gang member and pointed his gun at his sisters, pretending to shoot them. He expressed his heartbrokenness at witnessing what he took to be his own choices now influencing the behaviors of his own son. He also knew that his son was not the only one who had been paying attention; he had a reputation in the neighborhood, and he knew that a lot of children might be trying out the gang lifestyle. His hope was that, if he quit using, worked on his recovery, and became a better person, he could be a role model for others in his community. He saw this as the path for him to redeem himself and give a meaning to his life that he had yet to find. His family members listened and expressed their full support of his efforts at recovery.

Sometimes in addiction treatment reasons for change are not elicited so immediately (or powerfully!) from within the patient as they can be when they are first elicited from within the family itself. It is not only our experience but part of our knowledge that within families lie competencies and strengths which must be found and evoked as part of instigating movement within the patient himself. For

Scott, it might not have been enough for him to merely recognize he no longer wanted to be like other key figures he had known in his life. It was seeing (or re-seeing) what he wanted to be for his children and family through the inpatient sessions that allowed him to find within himself the aspirations to more fatherly and family-focused roles for himself: these reasons for change which were *evoked* from the family and then found within Scott himself were possible in the family setting in a way that might never have surfaced from an individual encounter with Scott alone. The power of evocation in the spirit of motivational engagement is augmented in family settings.

Working with Scott and his family gave me an in-depth look at the socio-cultural and environmental factors that predisposed him to heroin use and its impact on his family. This experience highlighted for me how much addiction is not just confined to individuals, but how it can deeply infiltrate and hurt communities and families. It also directed me to internally think about my own preconceived notions of who people are and who they can become. I think of several moments with Scott in which a less open stance towards him could have foreclosed his possibilities and held for all of us a less hopeful outcome. I also think how I would have felt less fulfilled by this experience had I shied away from more deeply engaging him with his family. It is so humbling to be a part of the process wherein Scott moved towards owning his behaviors and choosing what he would become in his future. Equally humbling is the acknowledgement of my own position in being merely able to meet him where he is as best as I can so that I can best facilitate the process that is Scott's: making the decisions about what life he wants for himself, his family, and his community.

Typical Concerns of Family Members About Co-Occurring Disorders

Family members and CSOs need emotional support as well as a better understanding of their loved one struggling with addiction or co-occurring psychiatric disorders during the process of treatment [26]. Providing psychoeducation about addiction, especially in the context of a psychiatric disorder, empowers families and loved ones. Key principles and topics of addictions that families benefit from learning about include:

- Specific DSM-5 diagnoses and the implications of these for the identified patient.
- Causes of co-occurring disorders and how substance use and psychiatric disorders affect one another.
- Types of treatment available for co-occurring disorders, length of treatment, expected outcome, and cost.
- Medications for both disorders.
- The role of the family in the recovery process.
- How treatment can help the family cope with their struggles.

- How the family can deal with some of the consequences of co-occurring disorders such as violence, suicidal behaviors, or relapse.
- Whether other family members are vulnerable to psychiatric illness, substance use, or both, especially offspring.
- When detoxification or inpatient treatment is needed.

Family-Based Interventions: What Works?

As discussed earlier, there is no evidence that family members exhibit greater personal pathology relative to the general population. Therefore, it makes sense for the clinician to always consider the family as a resource for helping the patient instead of a liability. A collaborative approach to working *with* (not on) the family emphasizes recognizing the suffering of the family and acknowledging its influence on the course of the addiction [27]. Family members should be conceptualized as change agents than rather adjunctive resources in the treatment process [27]. A five-step approach can lead to changes in coping, improvement in social support, and reduction in psychological and physical distress [28]. The five steps of the approach include:

1. Giving the family member(s) the opportunity to talk about the problem.
2. Providing education and information.
3. Exploring how the family member responds to their loved one's substance use.
4. Exploring, enhancing social support, and discussing the possibility of referral for specialized treatment.
5. Targeting improvements in couple's and family's functioning by any family-based intervention. In fact, "attention to the person's social context and support system is prominent among several of the most supported approaches [for alcohol use disorders] ([29], p. 276)."

Strong evidence exists that family involvement can help the person with substance use disorder to recognize the problem and engage in treatment [30]. Additionally, addiction treatment involving the individual's CSO results in more abstinence than does individual treatment [31]. Findings from research studies have shown that delaying conjoint or family intervention while the person focuses on individual recovery is not the right approach. Involving the family and CSOs early on in treatment can enhance treatment retention as well as improve treatment outcomes [32]. Specific clinical strategies include contingency contracting for treatment-related behaviors such as adherence to medications or attending counseling sessions; a focus on improving communication and problem-solving skills; improving interactions with family members and shared activities; and strengthening family members' skills to provide positive reinforcement for non-addictive behaviors and respond appropriately to drinking or drug use. Active case management strategies could be beneficial to help facilitate access to social networking and resources in the community. With adolescents, involving the parents or caregivers in treatment is extremely important and associated with better outcomes than providing individual therapy.

In our society, there is a myth that implies that family members and CSOs can do nothing if their loved one is not motivated to stop using. They may be told that they should wait for the person to "get ready" or detach from their loved one, hoping they will "hit bottom" and become motivated for change. There is strong evidence that an individual's motivation for changing substance use can be fostered by an intervention through CSOs, usually close family members such as a spouse and a parent. As discussed in a previous chapter, motivation for change is transactional, reflected in and affected by interpersonal interaction ([12], p. 140). As seen in the vignette of Scott and his family, the motivational power of *evocation* is amplified in its skilled use in family engagement.

A comparison of three distinct strategies for intervention through a parent, child, grandchild, sibling, spouse, or unmarried intimate partner to engage the unmotivated loved one in the treatment for alcohol problems was evaluated in a randomized trial [33]. One of these was the Al-Anon facilitation therapy which is designed to encourage involvement in the 12-step Al-Anon program. Al-Anon provides a mutual support for family members. Al-Anon does not endorse any theory of the etiology of addiction or family problems. Addiction is described as a "family disease" because of the negative impact on people who are close to the person with addiction. Al-Anon and Nar-Anon programs (for those whose loved one is involved in opioid use or other illicit drugs) advocate for self-care and "loving detachment" that encourage family members to avoid efforts to force the loved one to change and focus more on getting support from other members. Studies indicate that family members themselves do benefit from Al-Anon involvement, show decreased emotional and physical distress, and improve their coping [33].

Two other family interventions in addiction treatment were also evaluated alongside the Al-Anon program. The second intervention that was studied in the trial was pioneered by the Johnson Institute. In this program, CSOs are prepared for a confrontational meeting with the identified individual to trigger entry into treatment. The third intervention was a community reinforcement and family training (CRAFT) approach that teaches family members skills to avoid inadvertently reinforcing substance use behaviors and provide positive reinforcement for abstinence. CSOs are also trained in identifying windows of opportunity when their loved one shows more motivation for treatment and encouraging them to seek help. In brief, the results of the study suggest that the CRAFT approach was more effective in engaging unmotivated individuals in treatment (64%). The corresponding figures were 13% for Al-Anon facilitation therapy and 30% with the Johnson intervention. A consistent problem seen in previous reported aspects of the Johnson approach is that up to 80% of families find the confrontational approach unacceptable and refuse to go through with it. Among those families who decide to pursue it, however, most (75%) of their loved ones do enter treatment [33]. Other studies have demonstrated similar success rates with CRAFT among patients with drug use disorder [34, 35]. When family members and CSOs reach out to us reporting feeling helpless about what to do when their loved one is using drugs or drinking and is refusing to engage in treatment, we should be prepared to inform them about what intervention works the best, how to seek it out, and what to expect from it.

Unfortunately, there is little evidence for family therapy that includes children or involving the whole family unit in treatment. However, responding to the needs of *the most vulnerable* family members which are the children of parents who have substance use disorders should be a major focus in family-based interventions. Families can be helped to be more aware and understand the impact of addiction on children, examine how their own children may have been affected by the disorder, and work on reducing the impact in the future [36]. One key goal of family-centered addiction treatment includes engaging parents with substance use disorders to discuss openly with their children about the impact of substance use disorders on their family and the children. Family functioning can also improve with better communication, meals eaten together, and joint parent-child activities. Facilitating an evaluation of a child who exhibits any psychiatric or behavioral manifestations is warranted [36].

There is a major concern for many patients who have limited support systems or even no real family network. When some individuals seek help, some of these family ties may have already been destroyed and cannot be repaired. Therefore, no family members or CSOs exist who are willing to be involved in treatment. In such situations, one can work with the patients on establishing a social support system through the fellowship of 12-step programs and providing them with resources in the community through religious, spiritual and cultural pursuits, job training, and potential employment opportunities. A community reinforcement approach (CRA) focuses on connecting the individual with sources of positive reinforcement that do not involve substance use [37]. Peer support has been a key component of this approach. Involving the individual with peer support groups facilitated by peer workers who themselves are in recovery can be beneficial for patients with limited or no social support network.

I finish this chapter by sharing with you a reflective narrative about a family session from Jen, then a psychology intern, who had watched a powerful family session that I facilitated:

> *"Having seen a couple of your family sessions previously, I looked forward to the session and felt confident that it would be very therapeutic for Benjamin and his parents. At the same time, I felt more nervous about how it would go relative to other sessions I had seen you lead, given how strong Benjamin's defenses of presenting as overly competent and hard-working were, how much they had gotten in the way of him truly connecting to his experience and working on his recovery in the past, and how new it was that he had started to put his defenses aside and make real gains in treatment. When Benjamin came in holding a stack of workbooks and was initially futzing with the arrangement of the chairs, I had the thought, "here we go, he is trying to present as overly competent and like he has it all together rather than just listening and being open." However, I also had the thought that you would navigate that effectively and make sure it didn't get in the way, and looked forward to seeing how you would manage it. When Benjamin initially described what he had been struggling with and working on with his parents, I noted that he was long-winded, overly referred to the role of zolpidem (Ambien®, Sanofi-Aventis, Paris, France) in his actions and minimized the rest of his drug use, and seemed to want to show them that he had figured everything out and had it under control. I felt some slight irritation but also empathy*

at how hard this was for him and thought about the ways in which his defenses had likely been built so strongly as a way for him to cope with his feelings of insecurity, shame, and embarrassment about not managing his life well given how well his parents and siblings were doing in their lives. When you invited his mother to share her experience, I felt a lot of empathy for his parents and what they had been through, and again felt slight frustration tempered with empathy for Benjamin while he stared at the paper in front of him and intermittently jotted down notes about what his mother said. I felt relief when you invited Benjamin to put down his pen and just listen because I was eager for him to get past his façade and truly engage with the experience. I watched as Benjamin struggled with just listening to his mother and accepting the reality of his life and the impact on his parents. Although he interrupted her, I appreciated when you pointed this out and asked him to just listen. This seemed to make his mother feel validated, and it seemed that having the rest of the team in the room listening to his mother helped Benjamin realize that he needed to listen and face what she had to say at well. I felt some more relief as his interruptions became less frequent. When you asked his parents to think about what lines they would like to draw in supporting Benjamin and described the importance of clearly communicating that for enabling Benjamin to work on his recovery, I again felt relief that I think mirrored the relief that Benjamin and his parents felt. Even though it seemed like a difficult topic for them to broach and face, it also felt like it was important and empowering for them to see a path forward that would allow them to untangle themselves from the messes that Benjamin kept on creating and would enable him to take responsibility for his behaviors and their consequences. Your confidence while suggesting that they be thoughtful in establishing boundaries seemed to help Benjamin and his parents realize that his legal troubles were not insurmountable and for them to see, as a group, that this was the only path to build towards lasting change in his life. I noticed that, while it seemed scary for them, they also all disclosed a sense of relief and a new hope. When his parents thanked you profusely and communicated their appreciation for the session and Benjamin's care, I felt hopefulness for the family and a happiness that they could see a path forward that they wanted to follow-through on. I was also reminded yet again that, for so many patients with addiction and their families, the most important work of recovery is to fully confront the impact that addiction and mental health issues are having on the patient's life and those around them.

While this is difficult for patients and their CSOs to do, it is also imperative, as it empowers them to cope with the consequences of the behaviors and start taking steps to make changes and reclaim their lives."

References

1. Lewis C. The weight of glory. The essential CS Lewis. New York: Harper One; 1949.
2. Orford J. Empowering family and friends: a new approach to the secondary prevention of addiction. Drug Alcohol Rev. 1994;13(4):417–29.
3. Barnard M, McKeganey N. The impact of parental problem drug use on children: what is the problem and what can be done to help? Addiction. 2004;99(5):552–9.
4. Magill M, Apodaca TR, Barnett NP, Monti PM. The route to change: within-session predictors of change plan completion in a motivational interview. J Subst Abus Treat. 2010;38(3):299–305.
5. O'Farrell TJ, Fals-Stewart W. Behavioral couples therapy for alcoholism and drug abuse. New York: Guilford Press; 2006.
6. Barber JG, Crisp BR. The 'pressures to change' approach to working with the partners of heavy drinkers. Addiction. 1995;90(2):269–76.
7. Hunter-Reel D, McCrady B, Hildebrandt T. Emphasizing interpersonal factors: an extension of the Witkiewitz and Marlatt relapse model. Addiction. 2009;104(8):128–1290.

References

8. Edwards P, Harvey C, Whitehead PC. Wives of alcoholics: a critical review and analysis. Q J Stud Alcohol. 1973;34(1, Pt A):112–32.
9. Rotunda RJ, West L, O'Farrell TJ. Enabling behavior in a clinical sample of alcohol-dependent clients and their partners. J Subst Abus Treat. 2004;26(4):269–76.
10. Wegscheider-Cruse S. Co-dependency and dysfunctional family systems. In: Engs RC, editor. Women: alcohol and other drugs. Dubuque, IA: Kendall/Hunt; 1990. p. 157–63.
11. Woititz JG. Adult children of alcoholics. Alcohol Treat Q. 1984;1(1):71–99.
12. Miller WR, Forcehimes AA, Zweben A. Treating addiction: a guide for professionals. New York: Guilford Press; 2011.
13. Carruth B, Mendenhall W. Codependency: issues in treatment and recovery [special issue]. Alcohol Treat Q. 1989;6(1):200.
14. Hurcom C, Copello A, Orford J. The family and alcohol: effects of excessive drinking and conceptualizations of spouses over recent decades. Subst Use Misuse. 2000;35(4):473–502.
15. Miller WR, Hedrick KE, Taylor CA. Addictive behaviors and life problems before and after behavioral treatment of problem drinkers. Addict Behav. 1983;8(4):403–12.
16. Jackson JK. The adjustment of the family to the crisis of alcoholism. Q J Stud Alcohol. 1954;15:562–86.
17. Steinglass P. The alcoholic family: drinking problems in a family context. New York: Taylor & Francis; 1987.
18. Douaihy A, Daley DC. Substance use disorders. New York: Oxford University Press; 2014.
19. Meyers RJ, Wolfe BL. Get your loved one sober: alternatives to nagging, pleading, and threatening. Hazelden: Center City, MN; 2004.
20. Meyers RJ, Miller WR, Hill DE, Tonigan JS. Community reinforcement and family training (CRAFT): engaging unmotivated drug users in treatment. J Subst Abus. 1999;70:1182–5.
21. Orford J, Natera G, Copello A, et al. Coping with alcohol and drug problems: the experience of family members in three contrasting cultures. London: Routledge; 2005.
22. Gfroerer J, De La Rosa M. Protective and risk factors associated with drug use among Hispanic youth. J Addict Dis. 1993;12(2):87–107.
23. Moos RH, Billings AG. Conceptualizing and measuring coping resources and processes. In: Goldberger L, Breznitz S, editors. Handbook of stress: theoretical and clinical aspects. New York: Free Press; 1982. p. 212–30.
24. Velleman R, Orford J. The adult adjustment of offspring of parents with drinking problems. Br J Psychiatry. 1993;162:503–16.
25. Velleman R, Orford J. The importance of family discord in explaining childhood problems in the children of problem drinkers. Addict Res. 1993;1(1):39–57.
26. Daley DC, Thase ME. Dual disorders recovery counseling: integrated treatment for substance use and mental health disorders. 3rd ed. Independence, MO: Herald Publishing; 2004.
27. Copello A, Orford J. Addiction and the family: is it time for services to take notice of the evidence? Addiction. 2002;97(11):1361–3.
28. Copello A, Orford J, Velleman R, Templeton L, Krishnan MA. Methods for reducing alcohol and drug related family harm in non-specialist settings. J Ment Health. 2000;9(3):329–43.
29. Miller WR, Wilbourne PL. Mesa Grande: a methodological analysis of clinical trials of treatments for alcohol use disorders. Addiction. 2002;97(3):265–77.
30. Liddle HA. Family-based therapies for adolescent alcohol and drug use: research contributions and future research needs. Addiction. 2004;99(s2):76–92.
31. McCrady BS, Epstein EE. The theoretical bases of family approaches to substance abuse treatment. In: Rotgers F, Morgenstern J, Walters ST, editors. Treating substance abuse: theory and technique. New York: Guilford Press; 1996. p. 117–42.
32. McCrady BS, Epstein EE, Sell RD. Theoretical bases of family approaches to substance abuse treatment. In: Rotgers F, Morgenstern J, Walters ST, editors. Treating substance abuse: theory and technique. New York: Guilford Press; 2003. p. 112–39.

33. Miller WR, Meyers RJ, Tonigan JS. Engaging the unmotivated in treatment for alcohol problems: a comparison of three strategies for intervention through family members. J Consult Clin Psychol. 1999;67(5):688.
34. Meyers RJ, Miller WR, Smith JE, Tonigan JS. A randomized trial of two methods for engaging treatment-refusing drug users through concerned significant others. J Consult Clin Psychol. 2002;70(5):1182.
35. Meyers RJ, Miller WR, Hill DE, Tonigan JS. Community reinforcement and family training (CRAFT): engaging unmotivated drug users in treatment. J Subst Abus. 1998;10(3):291–308.
36. Daley DC. Family and social aspects of substance use disorders and treatment. J Food Drug Anal. 2013;21(4):S73–6.
37. Meyers RJ, Miller WR. A community reinforcement approach to addiction treatment. Cambridge, UK: Cambridge University Press; 2001.

Chapter 6
Spirituality, Religion, and Mutual Support Programs

> "What I really thought about was the result of many experiences with men of his kind. His craving for alcohol was the equivalent, on a low level, of the spiritual thirst of our being for wholeness expressed in medieval language: the union with God.... Alcohol in Latin is spiritus, and you use the same word for the highest religious experience as well as for the most depraving poison. The helpful formula is: spiritus contra spiritum."
>
> —Carl Jung in a letter to Bill Wilson, AA Grapevine [1]

Introduction

There is a growing acceptance of the importance of religion and spirituality in the treatment of addiction. As research on spirituality and addiction has been evolving, religious involvement remains one of the strongest protective factors in the prevention of alcohol and drug use initiation among children, adolescents, and adults, compared in size to family history [2, 3]. Religious organizations have been clearly shaping legislative policies related to primary prevention. People with substance use disorders tend to show low levels of involvement in religion and spirituality compared to the general U.S. population [4]. Involvement in AA, defined as a spiritual program, has been associated with abstinence [5]. Once abstinence from alcohol and drugs is initiated, religious involvement and recovery appear to have synergistic effect ([6], p. 267). Project MATCH, described later in this chapter, showed that religious/spiritual involvement increased after treatment and appeared to contribute to long-term abstinence [7]. Furthermore, over the course of recovery, spirituality tends to change and grow, as does interpersonal health [8].

Spirituality and Religion

Religion is defined as an organization that comprises a set of beliefs and traditions about some transcendent power in which its members have faith. Defining spirituality is more challenging. The origin of the word comes from Latin "breath" or "wind." It refers to the individual's personal experience of the sacred and its relationship to ultimate concerns like purpose and meaning in life, morality, suffering, and death [9]. Spiritual experiences transcend ordinary experiences. Spirituality may be connected or independent from a religious tradition. Spirituality has been operationalized and measured on multiple dimensions such as belief in a higher power, daily rituals of meditation/prayer, life purpose and goals, balance and wholeness, personal values (e.g., honesty, humility, compassion, forgiveness, and tolerance), and personal relationships [10]. From this perspective, people can identify themselves on a continuum of spirituality, being "less spiritual" or "more spiritual" along the various dimensions of spirituality [11].

Over 95% of U.S. residents report a particular belief in a spiritual dimension of reality [12]. In contrast, behavioral health clinicians, including psychiatrists and psychologists, are among the least religious groups in the U.S., and they may even have negative views about religion and spirituality which could make them reluctant to explore them in treatment [13]. Additionally, many U. S. treatment professionals who consider themselves enthusiastic about 12-step concepts rated spiritual change as unimportant in treatment [14].

Spiritual and Religious Treatments for Addiction

Longitudinal research has demonstrated that, once an individual is actively drinking or using substances, religious involvement (e.g., faith) is rarely sufficient to initiate the process of recovery. While faith-based addiction treatment programs are perceived by many as not offering real and evidence-based services ("pray away addiction"), the scientific evidence does not support this view [15]. A limited number of studies, including the Project MATCH (Twelve Step Facilitation arm of treatment), showed that spiritually-oriented addiction treatment programs perform at least as well as treatment programs with no religious or spiritual orientation. In one study, a Salvation Army program providing group therapy, job training, religious counseling, and AA meetings for "skid row alcoholics" was evaluated. This combination of interventions was compared to that of a halfway house and a hospital-based program treating the same population. After treatment, patients' alcohol use decreased by more than 50% and their employment rate increased by 55% when their treatment had some spiritual or religious component as above. Similar outcomes were seen with the comparison programs [16]. Another study demonstrated that patients treated in 12-step-oriented programs showed higher abstinence rates compared to patients treated in cognitive-behavioral-oriented programs 1 year after treatment

[17]. When the connection between spirituality and recovery was evaluated, spirituality was found to reduce the risk of relapse by serving as a protective buffer against the stress of early recovery [18]. In the same study, as recovery progressed, a spiritual orientation towards recovery was found to increase [19].

Mindfulness or transcendental meditation has been well demonstrated to decrease substance use among patients in addiction treatment and in the general population [20]. Mindfulness meditation is rooted in Buddhist *Vipassana* (translated as "insight") and encourages the cultivation of moment-to-moment awareness [21]. Although derived from Buddhism, mindfulness is secular in nature and open to any religious affiliation or none. Its practice is not necessarily spiritual, although it can be integrated into treatment with a spiritual component [21]. The compatibility of Buddhist mindfulness and 12-step programs was described incisively by Griffin [22], who reported practicing both approaches:

"Their (Buddhist mindfulness and 12 steps) respective means seem very different at times.... But I found that, as I learned more about both traditions, the deeper means and purposes of such came into harmony: understanding powerlessness helps me let go in my meditation practices; investigating my mind in meditation helps me do inventory work; listening to the suffering of others in self-help groups develops my heart of compassion." (pp. xviii–xvx)

Practical Considerations for Healthcare Practitioners About Spirituality and Addiction

1. Assess and explore religious/spiritual beliefs and core themes described by Paul Pruyser (1976) (including Awareness of the sacred, Providence, Faith, Gratitude, Repentance, Connection, and Vocation) [23] as fundamental aspects of the therapeutic process. Other practical approaches to assessing spirituality are discussed by Kurtz and Ketcham [24] in *The Spirituality of Imperfection; Storytelling and the Search for Meaning*. An effective tool, Values Card Sort [23] can help a healthcare practitioner better understand patients' strengths, hopes, and core values that define them.
2. Work with the patients on constructing a recovery-enhancing narrative of their life [25].
3. Encourage the patients while in treatment to engage potentially in 12-step programs and review their benefits for them, their family members, and CSOs.
4. Encourage involvement in mindfulness meditation and discuss its benefits.
5. Be involved in learning more about the role of spirituality/religion in addiction and recovery and how to better address it in your work with patients. Religious and spiritual leaders can, in turn, considerably benefit from learning about addiction, recovery, and collaborating with mental health practitioners.

The role of religion and spirituality for many of the patients we treat is a strong intrapersonal resource to draw on and evoke in the process of instigating recovery. For some people struggling in recovery, the religious or spiritual meaning of one's struggle could be the key thread which binds together a recovery narrative. While this dimension of a patient's life can be overlooked in the assessment of a patient's values and beliefs, experience and evidence both suggest it is a powerful part of a patient's beliefs that can be evoked and mobilized from within as part of aiding or instigating change. Even if a patient does not particularly espouse a body of spiritual beliefs in a religious sense, various spiritual practices exist in part as mindfulness techniques which the patient can be guided to master in the service of self-regulation and recovery.

Mutual Support Programs

The term "mutual support groups or programs (MSPs) or mutual help groups" describes a social network providing resources to support recovery. It includes people who are themselves in or seeking recovery and willing to help others who struggle with addictions. The old term "self-help" which was used in reference for such groups does not emphasize the reciprocal support, and, therefore, it is not accurate any longer. These programs are not considered as "treatment" or a "therapy" approach. They are considered an alternative approach to addiction treatment and a way of being and living. A significant number of outcome studies have evaluated the largest and most popular MSPs, which are based on the 12-step organizations. The focus of our discussion will be on the 12-step programs with an emphasis on the historical and research background of Alcoholics Anonymous (AA). It will help healthcare practitioners working with people with addictions differentiate between the distorted antithetical beliefs and views about AA and the core AA precepts and philosophy. I strongly believe that my appreciation of the impact of AA developed through attending AA meetings throughout my career; there is no substitute for it.

The Varieties of Mutual Support Programs

One way of understanding the different types of MSPs is based on the dimensions and philosophies that they promote [26]:

- Most programs are for people suffering from addictions. Others such as Al-Anon, Nar-Anon, Alateen are for family members and CSOs affected by a loved one's addiction.
- The focus is on the particular addictive behavior such as alcohol, cocaine, or opioid use, and behavioral addictions such as gambling or overeating.
- Particular beliefs and practices differentiate some MSPs. Twelve-step programs are explicitly spiritual in nature, whereas other MSPs—such as Secular Organizations for Sobriety (SOS) and Self-Management and Recovery Training (SMART)—are more secular in nature. The practice of SOS is like the 12-step

programs (mutual support) but separates the concept of sobriety from spirituality. SMART is a secular non-profit organization that offers both face-to-face meetings and online teaching of a combination of CBT and rational-emotive coping skills.
- Some MSPs (such as SMART and Women for Sobriety) use trained volunteer leaders, and this is prohibited in 12-step programs. Women for Sobriety is an abstinence-based, secular program with meetings facilitated by trained volunteers.
- Some MSPs, such as 12-step programs, promote lifelong fellowship, whereas others, such as SMART, are more time limited and not long-term support groups.
- Some MSPs—such as Moderation Management (MM) and Drink-watchers—focus on moderation versus full abstinence, whereas others, such as 12-step programs, emphasize full and lifelong abstinence. MM is the only alcohol MSP that addresses nondependent problem drinkers and considers moderation as an option.
- Some MSPs, such as Women for Sobriety, focus on empowerment and strengthening self-confidence, whereas others, such as 12-step programs, focus on accepting one's powerlessness, humility, and addressing problematic levels of self-focus and self-centeredness.

There is a *lack* of scientific evidence for the efficacy of these programs except for 12-step programs [27].

12-Step Programs

Worldwide membership in 12-step organizations is probably around 5–7 million people, with a significant number of those members living in the United States and Canada. Beyond AA itself, there are at least a dozen of other 12-step groups based on the same practices and views including Narcotics Anonymous (NA), Cocaine Anonymous (CA), Crystal Meth Anonymous (CMA), and Gamblers Anonymous (GA).

Bill Wilson—aka as Bill W.—and the two men who had a significant impact on him before he achieved sobriety had experienced a sense of existential transformation. In 1931, Carl Jung communicated with Bill W. that an American "alcoholic" named Rowland H. had sought treatment from him. He worked with Jung for almost a year and did well. He soon started using again, however, and reconnected with Jung. Bill W. [28] later acknowledged to Jung the importance of that return visit in the inception of AA, asserting:

> "*The conversation between you and Rowland that was to become the first link in the chain of events that led to the foundation of AA.... First of all, you frankly told him about his hopelessness, so far as any further medical or psychiatric treatment might be concerned. [Second, Jung answered his question about other hopeful treatments with the idea of] a spiritual or religious experience--in short, a genuine conversion.*" (pp. 26–27)

Because of his work with Jung, Rowland joined the Oxford Group, an evangelical organization, and stopped drinking. Rowland connected with his friend Ebby when he got back to New York and got him involved in meetings. Ebby, while visiting his friend Wilson, urged him to connect with "religion." Bill W. was not very accepting of the idea of replacing alcohol with religion. At the same time, he was intrigued by the spiritual transformation of Ebby through the Oxford Group and decided to explore what the organization was about. He was struggling with getting sober and conflicted about the existential issues of religion and God. He then admitted himself into treatment to address these issues while sobering up. While hospitalized, he experienced a moment of transcendence, his own spiritual awakening as he described it in 1957 [29]:

> "My depression deepened unbearably and finally it seemed to me as though I were at the very bottom of the pit. I still gagged badly on the notion of a Power greater than myself, but finally, just for the moment, the last vestige of my proud obstinacy was crushed. All at once I found myself crying out, "if there is a God, let Him show Himself! I am ready to do anything, anything!
>
> Suddenly the room lit up with a great white light. I was caught up into an ecstasy which there are no words to describe. It seemed to me, in the mind's eye, that I was on a mountain and that a wind not of air but of spirit was blowing. And then it burst upon me that I was a free man. Slowly the ecstasy subsided. I lay on the bed, but now for a time I was in another world, a new world of consciousness. All about me and through me there was a wonderful feeling of Presence, and I thought to myself, "So this is the God of the preachers!" A great peace stole over me, and I thought, "No matter how wrong things seem to be, they are all right. Things are all right with God and His world." (p. 63)

A few months later, after failed attempts by Wilson to convince other "alcoholics" to join the Oxford Group, he returned to Akron, Ohio, to his business. He struggled with urges to drink and made the decision to reach out to another "alcoholic" who was Dr. Bob Smith (aka Dr. Bob), a proctologist with a long history of drinking. They connected and discussed for hours and within few days Wilson moved into the Smiths' home for more conversations. Kurtz [30] recalled Dr. Bob's experience:

> "Yes, here was somebody who really knew how it was! This stranger from New York had 'been there.' He had felt the obsession of craving, the terrors of withdrawal, the self-hatred over failure--all the things that he himself, Dr. Robert Smith, had experienced and was experiencing even as he listened.
>
> Something happened within Bob.... [he had never talked about himself, to anyone. An only child, he had always felt isolated. He had always felt a] lonely pain of the deep conviction that no one else would or could ever understand....
>
> But there was someone who did understand, or perhaps at least could. This stranger from New York didn't ask questions and didn't preach; he offered no 'you must's' or even 'let us's.' He had simply told the dreary, but fascinating facts about himself, about his own drinking. And now as Wilson moved to stand up to end the conversation, he was actually thanking Dr. Smith for listening....
>
> 'I know now that I am not going to take a drink and I am grateful to you.' [Dr. Smith] had listened to Bill's story, and now, by God, this 'rum hound from New York' was going to listen to this. For the first time in his life, Dr. Bob Smith began to open his heart....." (p. 29)

Shortly after, Dr. Bob and Bill W. began their sobriety journey, and the initial foundations of the AA fellowship were established in 1935.

The two major components of the 12-step organizations are the *12-step program and the fellowship*. The program incorporates the 12 steps and 12 traditions. It focuses on abstinence and spiritual processes. Only the first of AA's 12-steps even mentions alcohol. Working the steps is sequential and involves the following spiritual processes: knowledge and relationship with God or Higher Power, making amends, openness to being changed, praying and meditating, self-searching, seeking God's will, and carrying the message to others [24]. Abstinence is conceptualized as the first step into the AA way of life, which is understood as a continuing journey towards wholeness and serenity [31]. The concept of God or Higher Power is intentionally flexible, and it emphasizes more the relationship with a transcendent presence [24]. In the AA beliefs, the core of "alcoholism" lies in *character* (not personality). AA described that "Selfishness-self-centeredness! That, we think, is the root of our troubles" [32]. Working and practicing ("in all our affairs") the 12 steps brings a recovery centered on spiritual growth.

The fellowship component of the 12-step programs involves the networking among members and sharing social activities. Having a sponsor is a major aspect of this fellowship. The sponsor is a person with experience in recovery and the program who provides support and guidance in working the steps. Twelve-step meetings may be either open or closed. Open meetings can be attended by anyone, and closed meetings are restricted for members with a desire to stop their addictive behaviors. The format of the meeting is either a step meeting, a speaker meeting sharing stories of addiction and recovery, or a discussion meeting.

Myths About 12-Step Programs

1. *AA is based on the disease model and does not encourage involvement in any other treatment approaches.* In fact, one way in which AA differs from the American disease model is asserting that it does not "take any particular medical point of view" [32], that "the main problem is in the mind rather than the body," and consistently describing "alcoholism" as an illness with many dimensions. It emphasizes the bio-psycho-socio-spiritual model. The AA book notes: "there is a solution," "there will have to be discussion of matters medical, psychiatric, social, and religious" ([7], p. 19). The approach of AA has been one of openness, inquiry, and allowance for differences [33].
2. *12-step programs promote pressuring and coercing people into it, even if they don't want to be involved.* The idea of externally coercing people to do *anything* has nothing to do with AA. The guidelines formulated by Wilson [29] for "working with others" (a similarity with the spirit of Motivational Interviewing!) are clear:

    "If he does not want to stop drinking, don't waste time trying to persuade them. You may spoil a later opportunity… if he does not want to see you, never force yourself upon him (p. 90)… Be careful not to brand him an alcoholic. Let him draw his own conclusions (p. 92)… he should not be pushed or prodded by you, his wife or his friends. If he is to find God, the desire must come from within." (p. 95)

AA members are encouraged to intervene in a supportive, listening, and non-confrontational manner as suggested by the Big Book. It is also clear that AA does not promote labeling people. Furthermore, the few clinical trials of coerced AA attendance have shown no benefits [34, 35].

3. *People who attend 12-step programs are pressured to discontinue their psychotropic medications.* The 12-step literature does not support this myth. Twelve-step involvement is compatible with adherence to prescribed psychotropic medications. At the same time, attendance has no negative impact on patients' attitudes towards adherence [36].
4. *The 12-step programs advocate the lack of responsibility for actions prior to sobriety, as it is articulated in the disease model.* AA, in contrast, advocates full moral responsibility and acceptance for one's own actions. In fact, in the fourth through seventh steps, members take responsibility by examining their past lives and recognizing their shortcomings (fourth step: *making a searching and fearless moral inventory*). In the eighth and ninth steps, this responsibility is focused on making amends for past actions. Additionally, Wilson has discussed his understanding of the "alcoholic's" power of choice: "As active alcoholics, we lost our ability to choose whether we would drink… Yet, we finally did make choices that brought about our recovery…. we chose to 'become willing' and no better choice did we ever make" ([29], p. 4).
5. *The 12-step programs only work for religious people.* Studies demonstrate that people's religious beliefs do not predict whether or not they benefit from the 12-step programs [37]. Atheists and agnostics are no less likely to benefit from these programs when they attend [38].
6. *There is no scientific evidence supporting AA's effectiveness.* There is a large and extensive research literature discussed below demonstrating the impact of AA on abstinence as well or even better than any other outpatient interventions.

Scientific Evidence for 12-Step Programs and 12-Step Treatments

There is clear evidence that attending more 12-step meetings is associated with lower level of addictive behaviors in the same or even subsequent period of time (first year, 3 years after treatment, and even 5 years and longer). The large number of studies involved AA and drinking outcomes [39–41]. More studies showed that AA attendance predicts long term sobriety apart from treatment [42]. One of the best outcome studies of AA showed that AA alone is not as effective as inpatient treatment combined with AA, particularly for patients with co-occurring alcohol and drug use disorders [27]. In addition, participation in AA predicts changes in spirituality, which in part contributes to the impact of AA on outcome [43]. An important point to emphasize is that the literature points to the concept of involvement beyond attendance in the 12-step program and fellowship. Besides the number of meetings attended, other aspects of AA involvement—such as having a sponsor, reaching out for help, and working through the first four steps—were significant predictors of positive outcome [44]. People who engage in high levels of altruistic behaviors such as supporting others in the recovery process are the most likely to achieve long term sobriety. Practicing the spiritual beliefs mostly benefits members. Regarding other outcomes such as self-esteem, anxiety, and depression, AA appears to have some benefit but not as much as it has on one's drinking. Research on drug-related 12-step programs is less comprehensive than research on AA. Positive findings on NA/CA are similar to those for AA [45, 46]. Participation in these programs predicted reduced anxiety, increased self-esteem, and decreased use of illicit drugs.

Involvement in treatment can help facilitate MSP attendance. Project MATCH designed and evaluated a 12 sessions of 12-step facilitation therapy approach (TSF). TSF is facilitated by a therapist, and its aim is to help patients to seek, find, attend, and get involved in AA as a long-term recovery program [47]. The project MATCH enrolled more than 1700 patients with alcohol use disorder who were randomly assigned to receive 12 sessions of TSF, 12 sessions of cognitive-behavioral therapy (CBT), or 4 sessions of motivational enhancement therapy (MET). All treatments produced excellent and equivalent outcomes [7]. Additionally, patients' outcomes were reasonably stable across 3 years of follow up. On one outcome measure, the percentage of patients who remained totally abstinent, the TSF group showed about 10% advantage compared to the other two treatments throughout the follow up. Furthermore, patients whose social networks do not support abstinence did better in TSF therapy only in the long run at 3-year follow-up which indicates that increased involvement in AA provided them with the support they needed. One additional finding is that patients with more severe alcohol use disorder did better in TSF therapy compared to CBT.

Practical Suggestions for Facilitating 12-Step Involvement

1. Use treatment as a window of motivational opportunity to encourage patients to be involved in 12-step programs.
2. Encourage patients to explore and sample many meetings and work on finding the safest, most welcoming, and supportive "home group."
3. Many people struggle to stay involved in 12-step programs. In the project MATCH study, 95% of those in TSF did attend AA during treatment, but only 41% of those no longer did so in 9 months [5]. Inviting patients to be involved in 12-step programs should be routinely and consistently done during treatment.
4. Discuss openly how 12-step programs work and review their core tenets and philosophy, especially the part about personal responsibility and choice, using the slogan "take what works and leave the rest."

Reflections from Clinical Practice

After Bill W. experienced his spiritual awakening, he was questioning its nature and meaning. He was wondering whether it was a hallucinatory experience or just a moment of transcendence and sublime truth. He then consulted with his physician,

Dr. Silkworth, who totally validated Wilson's experience and helped him believe in something of greater power than himself, something that was not alcohol: a transformative experience for Wilson, who never drank again. Since motivational factors may be more of an obstacle than aspects of 12-step philosophy and ideology, such as spirituality, my therapeutic approach has consistently integrated the elements of a "spiritual journey," as articulated by the patients working the 12-step program, with the motivational interviewing spirit, i.e., collaboration, evocation, and acceptance. Using motivational interviewing strategies explores the individual's ambivalence and commitment to give up alcohol or drug use and discusses 12-step involvement versus noninvolvement if one decides that stopping use is a goal. Furthermore, I focus my discussions with patients on helping them to develop personal responsibility for their behaviors and their impact on others, rebuild their value system, and strengthen and deepen a spiritual or transcendent—whichever was they define it—connection to others.

I have been challenged by many patients who refused to even consider attending some meetings because some AA Steps (Three, Five, Six, and Eleven) invoke God. As I understood, acknowledging "defects of character" and working on removing them are elements of the spiritual discovery. Refocusing the conversation on the concept of the Higher Power, which can be understood as any person/object that brings transformation and transcendence, and guiding the patients with interpreting the Higher Power as they see fit, the Higher Power can be anything they want. ("Made a decision to turn our will and our lives over to the care of God as we understood God."—Step Three.) Incorporating prayer and meditation into therapeutic work can considerably foster the transformational experience.

Kurtz [30] described how the core of AA philosophy is in conflict with some contemporary emphases on self-reliance:

> *"To the modern understanding, 'full maturity' means absolute, total dependence, and for the modern understanding, of course only full maturity is satisfactory… (to the AA way of thinking) human dependence…is not to be denied…To be human is to be dependent… Accepted ultimate dependence is the essence of the experience of bottom."* (p. 216)

In fact, AA "fellowship" encourages bonding with group members, which contributes to shifting one's social network and expanding it to others who support abstinence. It provides a sense of goal directness and strengthens socially healthy relationships. These behavior changes are active ingredients in 12-step programs processes and appear to contribute more to the positive benefits of 12-step mutual support groups than do 12-step specific factors or spiritual mechanisms [48]. Therefore, *depending* on these relationships is highly therapeutic.

A young woman told her story at the AA meeting in front of 50 members. She spoke of the desperation she had felt before recovery, of her sense of isolation and loneliness. When she came to her first meeting 3 years ago, she was surprised by the intensity of what she called the "bond" she felt with the people in the room: "I liked what I saw, and I've stayed ever since." She went on to talk about her recovery, about her loving relationship with her sponsor, and about her developing relationship with God. She ended her story by saying, "The biggest thing

I've gotten out of the program is my spirituality, my connection with God, because, "her voice trailing off as she continued, "because, you know, people disappoint…" ([49], p. 185).

References

1. Grapevine AA. The Bill W.-Carl Jung letters. New York: AA Grapevine; 1968.
2. Borders TF, Curran GM, Mattox R, Booth BM. Religiousness among at-risk drinkers: is it prospectively associated with the development or maintenance of an alcohol use disorder? J Stud Alcohol Drugs. 2010;71:136–42.
3. Miller WR. Researching the spiritual dimensions of alcohol and other drug problems. Addiction. 1998;93:979–90.
4. Hilton ME. The demographic distribution of drinking problems in 1984. In: Clark WB, Hilton ME, editors. Alcohol in America: drinking practices and problems. Albany: State University of New York Press; 1991. p. 87–101.
5. Tonigan JS, Connors GJ, Miller WR. Participation and involvement in Alcoholics Anonymous. In: Babor TF, Del Boca FK, editors. Treatment matching in alcoholism. Cambridge, UK: Cambridge University Press; 2003. p. 184–204.
6. Miller WR, Carroll KM. Rethinking substance abuse: what the science shows and what we should do about it. New York: Guilford Press; 2006.
7. Babor TF, Del Boca FK. Treatment matching in alcoholism. Cambridge, UK: Cambridge University Press; 2003.
8. Robinson EAR, Cranford JA, Webb JR, Brower KJ. Six months' changes in spirituality, religiousness, and heavy drinking in a treatment seeking sample. J Stud Alcohol Drugs. 2007;68:282–90.
9. Miller WR. Spirituality, treatment, and recovery. In: Galanter M, editor. Recent developments in alcoholism (Vol 16: Research on alcoholism treatment). New York: Plenum Press; 2003. p. 391–404.
10. Gorsuch RL, Miller WR. Measuring spirituality. In: Miller WR, editor. Integrating spirituality into treatment: resources for practitioners. Washington, DC: American Psychological Association; 1999. p. 47–64.
11. Miller WR, Thoresen CE. Spirituality, religion, and health: an emerging research field. Am Psychol. 2003;58:24–35.
12. Gallup GH Jr. The Gallup poll: public opinion 2001. Scholarly Resources: Wilmington, DE; 2001.
13. Miller WR. Integrating spirituality into treatment: resources for practitioners. Washington, DC: American Psychological Association; 1999.
14. Morgenstern J, McCrady BS. Cognitive processes and change in disease model treatment. In: McCrady BS, Miller WR, editors. Research on Alcoholics Anonymous: opportunities and alternatives. New Brunswick, NJ: Rutgers Center on Alcohol Studies; 1993. p. 153–66.
15. McCoy LK, Hermos JA, Bokhour BG, Frayne SM. Conceptual bases of Christian, faith-based substance abuse rehabilitation programs: qualitative analysis of staff interviews. Subst Abus. 2004;25(3):1–11.
16. Moos RH, Mehren B, Moos B. Evaluation of a salvation Army alcoholism treatment program. J Stud Alcohol. 1978;39(7):1267–75.
17. Humphreys K, Moos R. Can encouraging substance abuse patients to participate in self-help groups reduce demand for health care? A quasi-experimental study. Alcohol Clin Exp Res. 2001;25(5):711–6.
18. Laudet A, White W. An exploration of relapse patterns among former poly-substance users. Presented at the 132nd annual meeting of the Amer. Public Health Association: Washington, DC; 2004.

19. Laudet AB, Morgen K, White LW. The role of social supports, spirituality, religiousness, life meaning and affiliation with 12-step fellowships in quality of life satisfaction among individuals in recovery from alcohol and drug problems. Alcohol Treat Q. 2006;24(1–2):33–73.
20. Bowen S, Witkiewitz K, Dilworth TM, Chawla N, Simpson TL, Ostafin BD, et al. Mindfulness meditation and substance abuse in an incarcerated population. Psychol Addict Behav. 2006;20:343–7.
21. Hsu SH, Grow J, Marlatt GA. Mindfulness and addiction. Recent Dev Alcohol. 2008;18:229–50.
22. Griffin K. One breath at a time: Buddhism and the twelve steps. New York: St Martin's Press; 2004.
23. Miller WR, Forcehimes AA, Zweben A. Treating addiction: a guide for professionals. New York: Guilford Press; 2011.
24. Kurtz E, Ketchman K. The spirituality of imperfection. New York: Bantam Books; 1992.
25. White W, Laudet A. Life meaning as potential mediator of 12-step participation benefits on stable recovery from polysubstance use. In: 68th annual scientific meeting of the college on problems of drug dependence (CPDD); college on problems of drug dependence. 2006.
26. Nowinski J. Self-help groups for addictions. In: McCrady B, Epstein B, editors. Addictions: a comprehensive guide. New York: Oxford University Press; 1999. p. 328–46.
27. Humphreys K, Wing S, Mc Carty D, Chapel J, Gallant L, et al. Self-help organizations for alcohol and drug problems: towards evidence-based practice and policy. J Subst Abus Treat. 2004;26:151–8.
28. Wilson WG. The language of the heart. New York: The A.A. Grapevine, Inc.; 1988.
29. Wilson WG. As bill sees it: the A.A. way of life. New York: A. A. World Services; 1967.
30. Kurtz E. Not god: a history of alcoholics anonymous. Hazelden: Center City, MN; 1979.
31. Alcoholics Anonymous World Services. Alcoholics Anonymous. New York: Author; 1957.
32. Alcoholics Anonymous. Alcoholics Anonymous: the story of how many thousands of men and women have recovered from alcoholism. New York: Alcoholics Anonymous World Services; 1976.
33. Miller WR, Kurtz E. Models of alcoholism used in treatment: contrasting AA and other perspectives with which is often confused. J Stud Alcohol. 1994;55(2):159–66.
34. Walsh DC, Hingson RW, Merrigan DM, Morelock Levenson S, Cupples A, Heeren T, et al. A randomized trial of treatment options for alcohol-abusing workers. N Engl J Med. 1991;25:775–82.
35. Brandsma JM, Maultsby M, Welsh RJ. The outpatient treatment of alcoholism: a review and comparative study. Baltimore: University Park Press; 1980.
36. Tonigan JS, Kelly JF. Beliefs about AA and the use of medications: a comparison of three groups of AA-exposed alcohol-dependent persons. Alcohol Treat Q. 2004;22:67–78.
37. Conners GJ, Tonigan JS, Miller WR. Religiosity and responsiveness to alcoholism treatments. In: Longabaugh R, Wirtz PW, editors. Project MATCH hypotheses: results and causal chain, vol. 8. Bethesda, MD: National Institute on Alcoholism and Alcohol Abuse; 2001. p. 166–75.
38. Tonigan JS, Miller WR, Shermer C. Atheists, agonistics, and Alcoholics Anonymous. J Stud Alcohol. 2002;63:534–41.
39. Tonigan JS. Benefits of Alcoholics Anonymous attendance. Replication of findings between clinical research sites in project MATCH. Alcohol Treat Q. 2001;19:66–7.
40. Chi FW, Kaskutas LA, Sterling S, Campbell CI, Weisner C. Twelve-step affiliation and 3-year substance use outcomes among adolescents; social support and religious service attendance as potential mediators. Addiction. 2009;104(6):927–39.
41. Moos RH, Moos BS. Participation in treatment and Alcoholics Anonymous: a 16-year follow-up of initially untreated individuals. J Clin Psychol. 2006;62:735–50.
42. Moos RH, Moos BS. Paths of entry into Alcoholics Anonymous: consequences for participation and remission. Alcohol Clin Exp Res. 2005;29:1858–68.
43. Kelly JF, Stout RL, Magill M, Tonigan JS, Pagano ME. Spirituality in recovery: a lagged mediational analysis of Alcoholics Anonymous' principal theoretical mechanism of behavior change. Alcohol Clin Exp Res. 2011;35(3):454–63.

References

44. Tonigan JS, Rice SL. Is it beneficial to have an Alcoholics Anonymous sponsor? Psychol Addict Behav. 2010;24(3):397–403.
45. Gossop M, Stewart D, Marsden J. Attendance at Narcotics Anonymous and Alcoholics Anonymous meetings, frequency of attendance, and substance use outcomes after residential treatment for drug dependence: a 5-year follow-up study. Addiction. 2007;103:119–25.
46. Toumbourou JW, Hamilton M, U'Ren A, Stevens-Jones P, Storey G. Narcotics Anonymous participation and changes in substance use and social support. J Subst Abus Treat. 2002;23:61–6.
47. Nowinsky J, Baker S. The twelve-step facilitation handbook: a systematic approach to early recovery from alcoholism and addiction. San Francisco: Jossey Bass; 1998.
48. Kelly JF, Hoeppner B, Stout RL, Pagano M. Determining the relative importance of the mechanisms of behavior change within Alcoholics Anonymous: a multiple mediator analysis. Addiction. 2012;107(2):289–99.
49. Walant KB. Creating the capacity for attachment: treating addictions and the alienated self. Nothvale, NJ: Jason Aronson Inc.; 1995.

Part III
On Teaching, Learning, and Meaning

When an ordinary man attains knowledge, he is a sage; when a sage attains understanding, he is an ordinary man.

—Thich Nhat Hanh

So far, we have explored how my attempts to cultivate fullness in my approach to practice—integrating emphatic therapeutic connections with science-based practices—have led to a meaningful and rewarding career. I have had the privilege to share profound experiences of human suffering, resilience, and healing. In Part III, I share another key part of my career: my work teaching and mentoring the next generation of healers as well as learning from them. Their reflections capture what I have learned from their process of self-discovery. Finally, I share how my career has transformed me, helping define my value system, and helping me find meaning in my life.

Chapter 7
Trainees' Reflections on Clinical and Personal Growth

> *"In a real sense all life is interrelated. All [people] are caught in an inescapable network of mutuality, tied in a single garment of destiny."*
>
> —Martin Luther King, JR

Introduction

Throughout my career, I made the effort and took pride in bringing first and foremost empathy and compassion into the addiction practice. One key path to cultivating my "mission" has been to help healthcare trainees and practitioners develop and hold on to their passion and curiosity about people's unique experiences during their struggles with addiction. I am continuously inspired by pioneers such as Dr. Miller and Dr. Marlatt who have profoundly influenced my approach to addiction. Sharing clinical work with my trainees prompts me to reconnect with my own humanity when I have at times become emotionally detached and numb. Such experiential moments have been epiphanies that continue to enrich my identity as an addiction psychiatrist. They make me see what values matter the most: humility, honesty, hope, and gratitude. When Ernie Kurtz, the historian as storyteller and healer, was asked about the essence of great teachers, he reflected:

> *"There has to be a fundamental honesty. The first honesty for any teacher, of course, is "I don't know." That is so difficult for some people, and people who cannot say those words should never go into teaching. Some people, including myself, got into teaching in the hopes that someday you will know everything. Someplace along the line, you have to embrace what you know and don't know. Teaching requires that basic honesty."*

The very best aspect of my career has been the medical trainees I have worked with and mentored during their clinical psychiatry rotation on the dual diagnosis unit. I hope I have done it and continue to do it with the motivational spirit of evocation: by calling out their own humanism and passion for working with people with addiction.

This chapter is a bouquet of unique and genuine reflective experiences from diverse trainees who share about their work on our dual diagnosis unit. I have asked them to share how their work with patients and families influenced them on both professional and personal levels. Most importantly, I wanted to know how they integrated these experiences of "doctoring" into their value system, humanity, and whole identity. Motivational Interviewing (MI) as the humanistic approach was at the core of their clinical experiences. What they shared with me was as moving as any moment we had together in our daily clinical work. The depth of their expression, the impact of the experiences on their minds and hearts, and the way they used MI and the humanistic framework had broader effects on them than I had expected. The trainees reported the ways MI not only changed their clinical practice but also their personal ways of being with others. They spontaneously shared how it influenced their political, social, and philosophical perspectives on our healthcare and legal systems as well as their attitudes towards the identity of the other, including, most sensitively, those aspects which touch upon our racial, ethnic, and gender differences. I share with you these deeply personal and revealing reflections.

Learning to Treat Addictions by Embracing the Spirit of MI: Jen Forsyth, 2016

> "Prior to working on the dual diagnosis unit, I felt like I had a strong foundation in evidence-based therapies for broad psychopathology. I'd worked with patients with depression, anxiety, bipolar disorder, schizophrenia, and borderline personality disorder using Cognitive-Behavioral Therapy (CBT), Dialectical Behavioral Therapy (DBT), Acceptance and Commitment Therapy (ACT), and psychodynamic-informed frameworks. While I'd heard excellent feedback about the training on the unit and was looking forward to working with a new population (i.e., patients with a primary substance use disorder) and learning new therapeutic approaches (i.e., MI, Relapse Prevention), in retrospect, I had no idea just how eye opening, rich, and important my experience would be.
>
> The world of the dual diagnosis unit was qualitatively different from any clinical experience I'd had previously. Not only was it new to learn about the medical side of treatment (e.g., how withdrawal symptoms are monitored and treated), but I also found it eye-opening and incredibly powerful to see the world of patients with substance use disorders up close and to understand the broader systems that make many people vulnerable to developing substance use disorders (e.g., culture of substance use in certain occupational fields such as in physical labor to cope with physical pain; systemic issues of over-prescribing pain medications or sedatives in the medical field by practitioners who are not acutely aware of or trained in assessing for substance use disorders; transgenerational transmission of trauma and substance use to cope with painful emotions and situations; broad systems of psychosocial stress such as poverty and lack of resources or opportunities). I greatly value the knowledge I've gained in these areas as this has heightened my sensitivity to listening for and more thoroughly assessing for substance use issues in all clinical encounters I will have in the future. Understanding the common vicious cycle that many patients with substance use disorders get trapped in between using substances to cope with painful emotions that may or may not directly relate to co-occurring diagnoses, and then creating a worse situation for themselves while reducing their brain's capacity to cope with difficult feelings without impulsive actions has also heightened my understanding of how critical it is to

guide patients in taking a dualistic approach to treatment that targets both their substance use and underlying psychological pain.

Furthermore, learning MI in particular was a very different experience for me. While I now view MI as a treatment approach that easily complements CBT/DBT approaches to dealing with painful emotions and behavior patterns that perpetuate the problems in patients' lives, learning MI required me to unlearn some tendencies that stemmed from my CBT background. It also rapidly strengthened some broader clinical skills that I had focused on less in the past. I know these skills will make me a far more effective clinician moving forward. Some aspects of MI that initially felt at odds with my prior training but which I believe will be critical in my future work included learning to get to know a patient through open-ended questions. This skill helps patients communicate their story rather than trying to assess for specific symptoms or diagnoses. It also establishes a precedent for patients being active and thoughtful in their own treatment; I learned to trust that, if you ask evocative rather than closed-ended questions, patients will be able to tell you much more than you expect about the emotions and patterns that keep them stuck, about how they can move forward in effective ways, and frequently will 'talk themselves' into the changes they want to make. I learned to be much more comfortable with guiding patients to own the consequences of their actions and to reconnect with their painful emotions such as guilt, shame, and anxiety--the very feelings they want to avoid early on in treatment. I also became more adept at providing impactful and succinct reflections and summaries, and realized how powerful this was in helping patients change. Perhaps, most importantly, I became more comfortable in general with high acuity patients.

Overall, I feel like my experience learning MI on the unit truly rounded out my clinical experience and filled a gap in my training that was much larger than I realized. Given how pervasive substance use disorders are and how frequently patients minimize their substance use in other psychiatric settings, working on the unit has made me much more sensitive to potential substance use issues and much more comfortable providing effective treatment to a challenging population that, unfortunately, otherwise frequently receives insufficient or ineffective interventions. The specific MI tools that I learned will be helpful not only with patients who have substance use disorders, but will be helpful any time I am working with a patient who is struggling with ambivalence about what they want to change in their lives. Working with this population in the context of MI has helped me strengthen critical skills as a clinician more broadly, such as helping patients face painful emotions or consequences of their behaviors that they want to avoid, and learning to be precise and effective in my language as a clinician. My training in MI on the dual diagnosis unit has been one of my most fulfilling experiences, and I am truly grateful for it."

Humanizing Practice Through MI as a Means of Clinical and Personal Transformation: Isaac Petersen, 2016

"As a clinical psychology intern, I was slotted to complete a 3-month rotation in the dual diagnosis unit. My primary clinical background was working with children and their families, and I was intimidated by the idea of working with individuals with addiction co-occurring with severe mental illness. Moreover, I had never worked in an inpatient hospital before, so I was also nervous about working with such a challenging population in an intense, acute stabilization setting. How was I supposed to engage a patient in moments when previously building such an alliance with a patient took weeks and months? It was also unclear to me how relevant the training experiences would be to my future clinical work with children/parents and to my career.

Unexpectedly, the training experience in MI was the most valuable of my clinical psychology internship. It changed how I conceptualize and conduct therapy with all populations. It changed my perspective on interpersonal interactions and the challenging process of behavior change. I was surprised by how I was able to use MI skills to quickly establish rapport with challenging patients and to facilitate powerful interventions for change in the context of brief clinical encounters. I wondered how I had ever practiced before without the full complement of MI skills and spirit. In my three months on the unit, MI skills enabled me to guide severely depressed, suicidal, and substance-using patients to make positive changes in their lives, even in stays as short as a few days.

I learned more in this rotation than I did in any other. I grew more as a clinician and person in this rotation than any other. I learned MI skills that are relevant to all clinical (and non-clinical) encounters including how to: connect with people; use active listening techniques; give effective reflections; treat people with autonomy; and enhance people's motivation for change.

I am forever grateful for the invaluable supervision and training I received from the interdisciplinary team. I fully realized that MI is not just a "therapy"---it's a way of seeing the world and others. I now see therapy and interactions with people, more generally, in a very different way. My perspective, and particularly the MI one, will allow me to be more effective in all of the domains in which I work in which behavior change is the goal: whether as a therapist with children and families, as a research and clinical supervisor of trainees, as a course instructor, or in my day-to-day interactions with other people."

First Experience Learning to Work Therapeutically Using MI as a Way of Walking In-Step with the Patient: Erin Smith, 2012

"*Working with Jennifer was one of the most rewarding experiences of my rotation on our dual diagnosis unit. It was through our work together that I finally felt the MI style, employed with my own personal style, came together. This feeling was one of pure delight. It reminded me of the moment when, as a child, I was able to play my first piano piece in full, always moving the music forward even though some of the notes or tempos didn't come out exactly as I would have liked. This experience was even more gratifying when I saw Jennifer's surge in confidence and pride as she started mobilizing her recovery, progressing from an andante to a brilliant cadenza, guided by our work together.*

That being said, our first interview was an uncomfortable encounter: she apologized for crying yet expressed some of the most inspiring change talk I have heard ('I know I'm killing myself, but I want to live'). I squirmed in my seat, unsure of what to do with all this change talk and unsure how to engage someone who is sobbing and at her darkest hour. When reflecting on this, I realize that while I am armed and ready to 'roll with resistance,' I have tended to stop in my tracks within the face of such striking change talk. In my opinion, we as trainees are so relieved to hear a patient producing this language that we tend to stick with change talk and bask in its comforting glow. A shift in direction to commitment language is much more difficult; I was looking at change talk as an endpoint, whereas it reflects a patient's readiness, willingness, and ability to change, and is therefore only the beginning.

I brought about this change in direction by 'going deeper' with my reflective statements and taking risks in my hypotheses. Through these evocative statements, combined with open-ended questions aimed at being 'one step ahead of the patient,' I was able to elicit and strengthen Jennifer's motivation to change. This allowed Jennifer to discover more about herself and the life she wants. In doing so, her commitment language strengthened, and she started to take her first steps towards change. A particularly useful strategy was to make a reflective statement that touched on more painful, vivid content (thereby 'going deeper,'), and then follow this by asking how she felt in the present, how she was able to cope with this emotion, what she was doing differently, etc. Jennifer was also the first patient with whom I fully incorporated relapse prevention work as well as elements of other therapies, mainly CBT. These two points were extremely helpful in guiding Jennifer forward. I particularly enjoyed working on imagery with Jennifer, and we created shapes and colors for her emotions (e.g., a dense, black, shape-shifting cloud for anger), and she devised ways she could work through her emotions and visualize being in control of these powerful feelings (e.g., holding the now tangible emotion in her hands, throwing it out the window, replacing it with a small rainbow, etc.).

Our final session was bittersweet. I felt sad that our work together had come to an end, but also shared in Jennifer's pride and hope for her next chapter. 'I'm nervous and excited about transitioning to rehabilitation,' she said, 'at the same time, I know I can do it [stay sober, work her recovery,], I will do it,' she shared, beaming ear to ear. This was music to my ears and a testament to Jennifer's melody."

Humanistic Approach Using MI as a Vehicle for Advocacy for Patients: Brittany Atuahene, 2017

"When patients first arrive on the dual diagnosis unit, they are at a low point, the physical symptoms of withdrawal mixed with shame and guilt about their recent decisions. Each person is in a state of vulnerability, and, as the treatment team, we are expected to meet them in this space where they have as much spiritual discomfort as they have physical symptoms. I always struggled with the initial conversation. How can this encounter be therapeutic if the focus is on their drug use and the debilitating events which led to their hospital admission? Through the spirit of MI, change talk can be elicited by tapping into the patient's values. 'What do you believe keeps you alive?' is both a simple question and a turning point. It allows the patient to reflect on positive motivators in their life, a concept which many admitted they had not recently contemplated. My favorite part of the initial conversation with patients is reflecting on the fact that they made the decision to seek treatment. You can see a glimmer of hope in their eyes as they realize that they have made a crucial step forward: they see that their decision to seek treatment is all their own. You can see a spark of confidence. It is encouraging to witness that spark grow as patients spend more time on the unit. What astonished me the most was the drastic change between patients on the day of admission versus on discharge day! Some were hardly recognizable in both their appearance and words with which they spoke. It is no question that the person most surprised by the transformation was always the patient.

Working with patients with addictions was an inspiring and humbling experience. What I quickly learned was that the process had nothing to do with me. I had to be very conscious about the righting reflex (or known as the 'desire to fix'). My responsibility was not to 'cure' the patient, but help them find the space in which to explore their need for change. Through therapeutic work, each patient's potential was brought to light due to the work they accomplished while on the unit. Hard work pays off, and I was reminded of this with each of my patients.

What was so refreshing about working with our team was the example we set on how to treat patients with respect. If the patient was willing to put in the work and engage in treatment, then his/her presence on the unit was not questioned. It did not matter what was written in the initial 'intake note.' It did not matter how other staff members perceived the patient's situation. Every patient was given the chance to begin the work of recovery. There were many times when it seemed as if the patient had heard 'you can't' all his/her life, and I learned from my team to tell them 'you can.' When I think about my future career as a physician, I want to be that person for all of my patients.

One of the reasons I decided to pursue medicine was to become an advocate for patients. As I reflect on each of the patients I followed while rotating on the dual diagnosis unit, I can recount situations in which I had to campaign on their behalf. 'It is a possibility that John is here for secondary gain, but he needs his Electroconvulsive Therapy before we discharge him.' 'Linda is not just wasting our time. She is making progress. When you simplify concepts for her, she understands better.' 'Mary is not manic. She has some features of an eccentric personality style.' I was willing to speak up for these patients because I had taken the time to get to know them instead of passing judgment. It is amazing how well you can get to know a person in a short period when you put in the effort."

Humanistic Approach as Means of Empathic Connection Between Different Walks of Life: Emilie Transue, 2017

"As a trainee raised in an environment of privilege, I have been afraid of failing patients, being unable to accurately understand and empathize with their traumas, disparate backgrounds, and cultural idiosyncrasies, while scrambling to keep up with the extraordinary amount of medications and procedures available to confront illness. Wishing to bridge the gap, I ethnographically forayed into the experience of the 'other': reading books, watching documentaries, attending lectures. While I think this helped, it did not fast track me into producing authentic connections. Identity politics are complex: it is impossible to be fully versed in every magical combination of human uniqueness. Besides, there is no singular human experience, even other white girls from the suburbs experience vastly different lives.

After exploring this 'otherness' with patients, I have no doubt that societal stigma and pervasive misrepresentation are just as harmful as command hallucinations. Our dominant cultural narratives have a great inclination towards misrecognition, cutting corners with damaging stereotypes, tropes, and bias. They have become familiar daily anthems: women are weak, black is not beautiful, mental illness means weakness, substance use problems are simply a lack of a strong moral compass. For people like Devon and Keisha, these intersecting misrepresentations erased their personhood and all the accompanying unalienable rights to life and health.

Devon had been homeless for months, suffocating under depression, substance use, and a failing heart. After overdosing on whatever substances available, he was resuscitated, checked out in an emergency room, and returned to his original demeaning circumstances. Fortunately, Devon re-encountered his rescuing paramedic who convinced him to advocate for treatment. This paramedic, a saint of the streets, recognized Devon's humanity and his right to be healthy. Her insistence and encouragement refuted the voices misrepresenting Devon as a worthless, corrupt, and inferior leech on society. To this large, adult African American male, she had said 'your black life matters,' and now he was alive in our hospital chair, rediscovering the joy of pride and self-respect.

Keisha had known her HIV positive status for many years, but time had not dimmed the feeling of being tainted and unworthy. Years of alcohol, cocaine, and heroin use had been of little help either. As a woman of color, Keisha was expected to be the Strong Black Woman, forever giving and nurturing, irrespective of how her HIV status was a daily manifestation of a partner's betrayal, how it drowned her in rage and shame, and how it created a formidable barrier to intimacy. I had spent a lot of time with Keisha (my trainee status affording), and we explored her devaluing internal and external narratives. Ultimately,

Keisha reclaimed her image of a Strong Black Woman, rebelling against the oppressions of misrecognition. Gender, race, HIV status, and all, she said, let's start by loving me.

I have yet to meet someone who, at their core, does not want to be accepted for who they are. However, the absence of social recognition and affirmation is obstructive to health and wellness. Misrepresentations often compound on each other; it is no coincidence that my patients were people of color of low socioeconomic status. While I demographically belong to historical oppressors, Keisha and Devon exemplified that I do not need PhDs in their lived experiences to begin reparations. My act of sitting there, completely present in their self-expression, is recognition of their personhood, their right to receive treatment and to be well. Irrespective of the day and age, accurate recognition of the self is the basis of authentic connection and community. It is the greatest gift and 'treatment' I can provide. For in the end, what is more therapeutic than being recognized and loved for who you are?"

MI as a Way to Replenish One's Personal (and Clinical!) Spirit: Lauren Goldshen, 2017

"Throughout the first two years of medical school, I had a strong notion that I wanted to go into psychiatry. Despite the many appealing aspects of psychiatry, I remained hesitant because of my fear that bearing witness to my patients' emotional pain would take a toll on my own mental health.

Halfway through my third year of medical school I have a new, healthier, perspective on psychiatry after learning motivational interviewing. It was a false notion that my mental health is dependent on my patients' ability to change their own behavior; rather, it is related to my own sense of engagement with the patient. MI has helped me find a profound sense of professional and personal satisfaction on my psychiatry rotation.

In retrospect, I felt the most unfulfilled and burdened on other rotations when neither I nor my attending physician knew MI. I look back on unsuccessful attempts to change patient behavior: a surgeon giving a patient with lung cancer an 800-QUIT NOW card to 'counsel' him on tobacco cessation, or scolding parents for providing poor quality food for their obese children. This paternalistic technique benefited neither the patients nor us. Obviously, the patient who smoked knew smoking was harmful; after all, he was diagnosed with lung cancer. And clearly the parents in the pediatrician's office were aware of the effects of their unhealthy lifestyle as their daughters were morbidly obese and diabetic. Lecturing the patients only reinforced the problematic medical hierarchy and failed to consider the complicated circumstances behind these choices. Furthermore, it left us, the healthcare practitioners, with doubt that the patients would make changes because we never engaged them. We decided they needed to change, and we decided the correct solution for them without ever understanding their values or beliefs. We had set our patients up for failure and ourselves up for resentment and a sense of inadequacy.

Engaging patients with MI is truly a game-changer. MI is a two-way conversation where the role of the healthcare practitioner is to elicit and build on change talk from the patient. It relieves the practitioner of the burden to force change on the patient and allows the patient to be a true partner in their care. When a patient is reluctant to change, I respect their ambivalence because I have engaged the patient and I understand more about the roots and circumstances of that behavior.

At the same time, MI also removes the credit that healthcare practitioners feel they 'deserve' from the patient's success in behavior modification. My first patient was Tiffany, a woman with a 10-year history of not using substances and being in recovery. After losing her house and belongings to a fire and with her boyfriend going to jail, Tiffany spent her remaining $8,000 on a month's worth of crack cocaine instead of finding new housing. In *our first few encounters, Tiffany could not get through a few sentences without crying about her past mistakes. I felt awkward because I wasn't eliciting enough change talk and we kept circling around her hopelessness, guilt, and embarrassment. I was tempted to respond, 'It will be okay' or, 'I know you can get through this.' Maybe those statements would've relieved me from the heaviness of the conversation, but coming from me, those remarks would not have reassured Tiffany.*

A major turning point occurred following an incident where Tiffany threatened to choke a staff member on the unit. When Tiffany entered our treatment team room, she announced with a huge smile, 'I am so proud of myself.' I was puzzled as I was expecting Tiffany to be remorseful or even irritated. Tiffany then explained that after her anger outburst, she apologized to every staff member and the patient that witnessed the event. She started crying and said, 'This is the first time I took accountability for anything in my life.' I felt vulnerable to surmise about such a personal matter, yet at the same time I replied by inquiring if there was a connection between controlling emotions and controlling the choice to use substances. Looking in Tiffany's tearful eyes, I knew this resonated with her. I asked Tiffany what it felt like to make a change in her usual behavior and she responded, 'freedom.' I stayed in the moment with Tiffany, and we explored how using substances was a frequent response to anger and something that Tiffany never felt was possible to control until this day."

The beauty in the humanistic approach to therapeutic work and particularly the MI spirit is that the hope and change truly come from within each individual patient. I can think of no other circumstance that would give me greater professional and personal satisfaction in medicine."

Humanistic Practice as Means to Self-Discovery: Jennifer Darby, 2017

"I cannot overstate how much I enjoyed my experience on the dual diagnosis unit. Although I learned a lot about many aspects of patient care, I think the most striking lessons were those I learned about myself. I see this self-discovery as integral to my medical education because I believe that feeling like a hypocrite as I counsel patients is somewhat antithetical to the therapeutic alliance. Here is a brief list of some of the most important lessons I took away from this rotation focused on working with patients with addictions:

1. *Personal responsibility. Fully embracing oneself as responsible for one's actions is the difference between working towards real change and treading water. Although it is tempting to blame auxiliary circumstances for behavioral choices, it is maladaptive because it prevents us from learning how to cope with a new situation in a healthy way. Taking ownership of behavior is the ONLY way to enact positive changes.*
2. *Language matters. I believe I have become a more effective communicator while saying the same thing by making more deliberate choices with the most automatic aspects of language: swapping out the parts of speech we never think about like "but" and "why" for phrases like "at the same time" and "what makes you." I have noticed the ways in which this facilitates further discussion.*
3. *Don't be afraid to ask. I have never shied away from difficult topics, but I now feel enormous confidence discussing even ridiculously sensitive things. For instance, I motivationally interviewed my mom about her ambivalence about seeing a therapist. This is something I've been encouraging her to do for years, but by exploring the reason that she was reluctant to do so and asking about her perspective, more progress was made in that direction than ever before.*

4. *Connect the dots.* More than ever, I am aware of the complicated tapestry that weaves together all the experiences and decisions that shape a person. Having a 'curious and itchy mind' means being willing to look at the full expanse of tapestry, not ignoring or shying away from certain parts because they are painful to see. Paying attention to the way things fit together is the most effective way to gaze upon the space between the things we naturally choose to look at, to see the things that we most need to see."

Person-Centered Approach as Supplement to Treating Serious Chronic Illnesses and Understanding the True Meaning of Empathy: M. Usama Hindiyeh, 2017

"Prior to my HIV Psychiatry elective rotation, I thought I had a respectable understanding of what empathy meant, what it looked and sounded like, and how to apply it in a clinical setting. My impression was that over my third-year rotations, the various medical teams I worked with were applying an empathic approach to care. However, over the course of this elective during which I learned about the motivational interviewing approach, I was inspired to reexamine what empathy truly means.

The HIV Psychiatry elective is a unique rotation in which fourth-year medical students split their time between the dual diagnosis inpatient unit and the HIV primary care clinic. With the rising use of intravenous opioids across the U.S., clinicians are facing a growing epidemic of opioid drug use and new HIV infections. During this elective, students are challenged to approach HIV care in a holistic manner and delve deeper into the co-morbid psychiatric illnesses among these patients. Moreover, they are challenged with the task of providing therapeutic sessions in which they try to establish a therapeutic alliance and work with patients to evoke behavioral changes in their health.

After a few days of approaching my care with the 'skills' or frankly the 'habits' I formed throughout my medical training, it became clear that my sessions with patients were going to be largely un-therapeutic or counter-therapeutic if I continued with my current method. Specifically, my approach, while initially started with one or two open-ended questions, quickly transitioned into narrow closed-ended questions. If patients displayed emotions, I would acknowledge them but redirect our conversation without exploring those emotions further. Moreover, I felt my goal or agenda was to provide 'expert advice' and specific treatments for the patient rather than develop the treatment plan with them. While my intentions were to genuinely help my patients, my method was practitioner-focused rather than patient-centered. At best, I was sympathetic when patients would share their experiences with me, but my responses lacked the empathy necessary to gain my patients' emotional trust. Especially in the treatment of addiction, the literature and my short experience on this rotation would suggest this approach will largely be unsuccessful.

After reading about MI and practicing its spirit and skills deliberately and repeatedly, I developed a new 'empathic spirit' towards providing care, which ultimately enriched my sessions into reflective and therapeutic experiences. The agenda of the sessions were largely patient-driven (i.e., 'What led you to seek treatment?'), and my role was to guide and inspire my patients to develop ways to evoke change. In this learning experience, the initial changes I made in my approach was staying consistent with open-ended questions and actively listening to my patient's responses and emotions so I could provide genuinely empathic reflections. With these initial changes, I quickly noticed a new therapeutic alliance developing between my patients and me. Additionally, the patients that were ready to make changes in their health could articulate their self-discovered motivations and plans for those changes.

So, what does empathy mean to me now? It means actively listening to another individual's experience and implanting yourself inside that experience, so you can reflect upon that experience with them. Caring for your patients and having good intentions are vital, but they are inadequate to be an effective clinician. One must adopt and apply the 'empathic spirit' of motivational interviewing if one hopes to inspire one's patients to make behavioral changes in their health."

Humanistic Practice as a Treatment for the Trainee's Soul

Alexandra Sansosti, 2017

"As I looked across the table, cold, sad eyes were the first things I saw. The tattoos of bones and initials along the perimeter of the jaw line I guessed had substantial significance, but of what? His hair was cut short, almost like the cut of a soldier, appearing hardened, like the bones inked on his collar. Ernie looked me right in the eye, 'I want to get better. This shit is taking my soul.' My attending AD repeated those words once he left. 'Alexandra, he just shared with you this amazing disclosure. Why did you not ask more about it?' Curious and itchy mind!!! (Stephen Rollnick, 2017)".

"Something was off, I thought. I learned within that moment that I had been off. Despite his outward appearance, Ernie had gentleness in the way he talked. Truthfully, I probably would have been startled by this patient had I encountered him walking down the street. But as I sat in his room talking with him, there was a dissonance between what he was telling me and his vulnerable tone. He elaborated on his tale of 'relapse': familiar yet exaggerated. He explained that he is a drug dealer and sells heroin. When he runs into financial trouble, he turns to selling drugs because he says, 'I know I can make about $45,000 in a week.' He added a half-hearted, 'I'm really not a big deal though in the scene, you know?' Perhaps he said this because of the slightly prolonged silence or the terrible poker face I was trying to keep.

He described a life of slavery to the drug: when he begins to sell; he starts getting high; he gets into trouble or comes into the hospital to detox; repeat. He painfully told me with tears in his eyes that his girlfriend is on her way to inpatient rehab today, and that he is crushed by the responsibility of having introduced and exposed her to heroin. He feels remorse about his kids, whom he described as 'amazing,' but whom he has let down one too many times. And, finally, he said to me, 'but the thing I feel most terrible about is when I'm in that Motel 6 bagging 1,500 bundles thinking about all the families this will tear apart, all the lives it will take, and all of the sadness this will bring.

I worked with Ernie for the next few days. His words and demeanor bore all the stigmata of true intrinsic motivation for change. He was engaged, interactive, diligent, and always came to treatment team with new reflections on what we had discussed the day previous. I hadn't seen many patients, but I was impressed with the initiative that he demonstrated. On a Thursday afternoon, I came to talk with him on my own and he asked me if he would be able to be discharged the following day. He told me that he had been thinking about his outpatient treatment and that he wanted to go to the methadone clinic. He didn't feel it was so productive to stay over the weekend to complete the last day of his detoxification taper just to leave and go to the methadone clinic. He reasoned through with me that he knew himself and would need the support of the clinic to keep him honest and to work his recovery at a reasonable pace. The attending psychiatrist agreed with his proposed plan. Ernie was set to leave the next morning after treatment team.

The following morning, we began seeing the new patients and planned to see Ernie before his discharge. At some point during the morning, my attending received a text message from one of the other clinicians that said, 'The Federal Marshal is here for Ernie.' We were shocked. Had he mentioned legal charges? No, everyone agreed they had heard nothing from him regarding legal charges. The social worker verified that she had asked him if he had a parole officer and he had said no. What could this be then? What was happening? How could this patient, so motivated to get into recovery, possibly be in this situation, so close to the start of his journey?

I walked into the treatment team room to find out why the Marshal was here: violation of parole [by coming into the hospital and seeking addiction treatment] after imprisonment for aggravated assault, attempted homicide, possession, distribution.... The list continued. I said nothing. I knew this person. I knew he wasn't "a bad person", and, regardless, I knew he wanted help. He was genuine in his intent to get better. He wanted to move on and have a better life for himself.

I told the other clinicians that we would still need to see him before he left to make sure he had the medications that he needed and all the resources to get connected back to treatment when he was released from prison. I returned to the rounding room with a whirring pool of emotions that I attempted to sort out while the resident interviewed the remaining few patients.

AD gave me the signal to go get Ernie and told me that he would help with the interview, as he was not sure if the patient knew he was going to be discharged to prison. When I arrived at the patient's room, he was gone. 'Where the hell did Ernie go?' I asked one of the other clinicians.

'We are so sorry, Alexandra; the Marshal would not wait. Security told him and he silently walked off the unit. There was no fuss. He just left a little while ago.' I could feel the stinging tears and the rising anger that was building inside of me. He was a patient. A human patient. And we had deprived him of his ability to be successful in the long run. We had fed into the system of punishing those who are at the bottom. And we had deprived him of adequate medical care.

I was glad that I had the opportunity to get to know Ernie before I knew about his charges. In a way that he probably did not recognize, he gave me a wonderful gift. I would have likely judged him early on had he told me what he had served jail time for. But the reality is that good people do bad things. And regardless of the determination of whether a patient is "good or bad", all patients deserve our attention, our care, and, at those things, our very best. We do not pick and choose the patients that we treat; we treat them indiscriminately.

I find that I derive my opinions from experience, and this experience that Ernie gave to me has certainly informed one of my perspectives. Our patients should feel safe coming into the hospital. Health is not connected to the justice of legal disposition. This patient was not given the opportunity to obtain his medications, get counseling, say goodbye to his doctors, or have any sense of closure for his care. I was unable to send his medications to the prison because the Marshal did not specify which federal prison at which he was going to be held. He will likely hold resentment towards the medical system, refrain from seeking treatment in the future, and quite possibly is already shooting heroin into his veins as I write this reflection. I hope not. But everyone who told him he could do it did not even afford him the simple courtesy of saying goodbye."

When will we recognize that punishing those who come to seek help returns reward to no one?"

Shriya Kaneriya, 2017

Shriya, a third-year medical student who rotated on the dual diagnosis unit, described her clinical experience with Chris: "humbling and transformational." I hope it might provoke you to reflect on your own clinical work and how it shapes your life, your values, and your relationships. And I hope that it pierces through all medical mantles (including all white coats) and resonates within you on the most human of levels. There have been moments of astonishment when patients have uttered spontaneously to me truths about themselves from the deepest reaches of their souls in ways I surmised were unprecedented for them. It is another experience entirely to have a trainee capture these moments of authenticity in such detail while revealing the intimate nature of the trainees' own internal processes, vulnerabilities, and uncertainties. I have struggled within myself over stretches of time to articulate the meaning of these clinical, personal moments in the most powerful encounters I have had with patients. Still, I have not been able to capture in words any experience that I have had in the way this trainee has. I am so grateful to have been privileged to receive this written moment from Shriya in an experience that was so moving for me on the clinical floor but took on new dimensions when she shared it with me in these words. It is with the same hope that she beautifully describes that I share it with you, hoping that you are moved within yourself the way I have been moved by this reflection written in the clearest but most unassuming of ways about the most genuine of clinical moments.

> *"I read his chart before having my first engagement session with Chris on the unit: A 50-year-old man presenting with suicidal ideation, aborted suicide attempt with heroin and cocaine overdose, homicidal ideation of driving his girlfriend off a cliff, and a history of imprisonment. His presentation couldn't have been more different from the life I've lived and known. I didn't know what to expect or how he would receive my presence. There was a part of me that was nervous about how I would be able to connect with him.*
>
> *When he walked into the room, he appeared disheveled, tired, and with poor dentition. He had partially visible tattoos up both his arms. He was irritable and closed off, responding in vague terms and talking about people 'pissing me off' and his just being 'done with it!' I could tell he was making efforts to stay superficially polite on top of the simmering rage kept inside the wall he built around himself. I had trouble empathizing because I felt disconnected and confused about his sincerity.*
>
> *It was in our second full session together that something incredible happened to shift the dynamic of our relationship. There came a moment when he, in words he later shared, unburdened the darkest parts of his soul. He spoke about having tried so many times to stop using drugs, including rehabs, NA meetings, outpatient programs, but always hitting a barrier at a particular step. He was devastated at not being able to reconcile the broken relationship with his daughter. He felt shame, guilt, resentment, and frustration about her having knowledge of his behaviors and his series of ongoing failures. It was then that I experienced the difference between what it means to be there for someone and actually being there with them. Despite the presence of six other people sitting in on that conversation, for those moments it felt like it was just he and I. I was connected. We were connected. What took me aback was when he told me that in all his years struggling with recovery, he had never shared this information with anyone before. He appeared physically exhausted after sharing, yet noted that he was also overcome with relief. In the*

moment of silence after Chris walked out the room, I was overwhelmingly humbled by the fact that I suddenly knew more about this man than anyone else in his life, despite having met him just 24 hours ago.

Opening up about his daughter was a huge step forward for him. At the same time, it unleashed years of unresolved emotions, especially anger. He became emotionally dysregulated. At one meeting, he would be engaged in strong change talk. The next morning, I would come in to find out that he had punched a wall the previous night after an argument with his girlfriend at visiting hours. Five steps forward, three steps back. It was an emotional roller coaster. We worked together on anger management skills, coping strategies, and taking pauses to evaluate situations before responding. We discussed his tumultuous relationship with his girlfriend and the importance of focusing on himself and his recovery first. Working closely with Chris in therapy sessions challenged my own unconscious biases and the misguided morality often placed by society on addiction. It made me personally reflect on the way I deal with my own life problems and realize how we as healthcare professionals don't always take all the advice that we give.

We work with patients on strategies for appreciating emotions as transient waves as opposed to permanent states, yet we are sometimes quick in mental health care to make judgments on a person's character based on a single moment in time. We can stigmatize the very people we set out to treat. Every morning at treatment team, some staff would report Chris as 'irritable' with an underlying connotation of 'troublemaker' even though he had not been aggressive towards any of the patients on the floor. In practicing MI skills, I became more aware of labeling terminology such as 'deviant' and 'criminal,' and their negative impact on patient care. Yes, he was 'irritable' and safety concerns needed conveying: at the same time, I found myself advocating for him because I knew him to be more than just an 'irritable' man. I witnessed him reflecting on his behaviors, recognizing his mistakes and sharing anecdotes of how he was trying to better regulate his impulsivity on the unit. It wasn't fair to expect him to behave differently in only a few days. Recovery, much like life in general, is the willingness to commit oneself to a long-term journey. I found that when I could better understand his intention, I was able to make fairer evaluations of his behavior.

As I got to know Chris better, he became a real person to me, not just a diagnosis or a paragraph in his records. I learned that even though I might not be able to understand some of his thought process or impulsivity, I could empathize with someone from an entirely different walk of life if I took the time to truly listen. At first, I observed a man who was using drugs and was covered in tattoos. Later, I learned the story behind the tattoos, each arm a reminder of one of his two children. Whatever his past may have been, Chris was ultimately seeking what most every human being is seeking: family, home, human connection, to love and be loved. What he wanted was to reclaim himself, be the kind of father he used to be, be in a trusting relationship, and find sense of purpose and self-worth. These are all human needs deserving of attention and respect.

As I practiced embodying the spirit of MI and humanism in my patient sessions, I gradually became more aware of the influence of my own posture, facial expressions, and tone of voice and language on creating a safe space. In the process of evoking change talk, I had firsthand experience understanding the immense impact of various social determinants of health. The main key to Chris's recovery was not his diagnosis or medications; it was a commitment to behavioral change and managing psychosocial stressors. It was enlightening to experience patient care in a team-based approach, reach out to family members for collateral information, and work closely with the social worker to make sure his treatment didn't end when he stepped outside the hospital. I gained insight into the barriers unemployment, transportation, unstable housing and support system, chronic medical comorbidities, and lack of health insurance can place in front of an individual who is motivated to change. Because Chris did not have health insurance, the social worker had a difficult time finding rehab centers that would accept him and fit his needs. It was frustrating to *accept that, despite the patient finding great courage to keep working on his recovery, there were systemic limitations curbing progress.*

Additionally, I had to learn to cope with the emotional impact of sharing Chris's struggles and my desire for him to succeed in continued recovery outside of the hospital. A day before expected discharge, he wanted to sign himself out against medical advice after his girlfriend told him she threw all his belongings out of their house. The social worker was still working on setting up his aftercare at a rehab facility. Eventually, after talking with him about his concerns, he calmed down and decided to wait another day for aftercare to be arranged. I spoke with my team about the experience and worked on applying the 'Serenity Prayer' to the concept of patient autonomy. At the end of the day, the patient will leave the hospital and choose to do what he or she wishes to do. I learned to accept the difficult truth that I cannot help someone who does not wish to be helped. change is ultimately a choice one makes for on self.

Working with patients who are recovering from addiction has been an intimate experience with one of the most powerful human emotions, that of hope. Uncertainty, I appreciated, is a natural facet of hope. I've been moved and inspired by the resilience of patients like Chris. To have played even the slightest part in another's discovery of hope in a seemingly hopeless place has been a profound privilege."

Gil Hoftman, 2017

Another reflection which came from a very dedicated, caring psychiatry resident showed the spirit of MI as keeping a candle lit amidst the darkness of a patient who was losing hope for himself in ways he himself might not have been aware of or was able to articulate. The experience captured here exemplifies how the motivational element of hope (and its evocation) can be sparing for the practitioner even when the patient's reality is one in which hope has been lost. It shows powerfully how even in the face of the most abject of clinical realities, a motivational perspective does not promote flinching from such an experience, but it instead allows the practitioner to hold within himself the deep and painful realities of loss, hopelessness, and even the choice to end one's life.

"Like many people who commit to becoming medical doctors and healers, I have always wanted to help people recover from illness. But how could I transform that desire into action? I also wonder, how would I deal with a situation where I failed to help?

Far too often growing up in the U. S., I have been told that I control my destiny and that if I work hard I will succeed in whatever endeavor I choose. This is a wonderful, empowering, yet woefully incomplete perspective. I have learned that in contrast with this culture of individualism, I was fortunate to have influential mentors who modeled humanistic approaches and nurtured my development as a psychiatrist-scientist.

During my 4th year of medical school, after deciding I would pursue psychiatric specialization, I joined AD on the dual diagnosis unit for a sub-internship month. Immediately, the experience provided me a platform and language that transformed my desire to be a healer into action. Through the language of MI and the humanistic approach, I found a non-patronizing and emotionally-connected way to talk to people about their psychiatric illnesses. I have learned the theoretical background and practical skills, encouraging dynamic growth and thirst for curiosity. During medical school, there were no comparable rotations during which I had a wonderful team-bonding experience with resident physicians, psychology interns, pharmacists, social workers, case managers, and nursing staff all *supporting each other and committed to patient care. This team work and support, combined with a delicate balance of supervision and autonomy, truly fueled my internal passion to become a healer.*

I was fortunate enough to stay in Pittsburgh for my residency training and work for 2 more months on the same unit. One key experience during my internship occurred while working on the unit. I received a startling text message from one of my colleagues on a typical afternoon: 'Did you hear our shared patient died? He jumped off a bridge last night... I'm watching the local news...they identified his body.'

Ryan was only 28. He was under my care on the dual diagnosis unit for a week before being discharged. The team had assessed that he wasn't actively suicidal. Yet two days later, he died. What happened? Did I miss an important signal and make a poor decision to discharge him? Could I have done a better job?

Two weeks ago, Ryan was standing on the side of a bridge when the paramedics found him. He was high on opioids and contemplating jumping. Eventually, he was hospitalized for the third time in a month. His family relationships were badly damaged; he was poorly educated and unemployed, without an intimate partner, support group, cohesive identity, or purpose. He was kicked out of multiple homes and had legal charges pending. His life was shattered.

Ryan and I spent hours together discussing treatment options and trying to develop his motivation to stop using heroin. When sober, Ryan was introspective, respectful, and soft-spoken. Though he initially seemed encouraged, his motivation to change quickly faded while his urge to keep using heroin increased. After a few days, Ryan's goal was to leave and start using again.

Each day, I felt like I was falling short when trying to reach him: I was completely powerless against his opioid addiction. Though I spent considerable effort trying to engage Ryan, he remained aloof and disinterested. I wanted so much to alleviate his suffering with alternatives to opioids. He was convinced that medicines and psychotherapies were ineffective. I saw that opioids had damaged his life severely. He recognized heroin was dangerous but said it was worth the trouble. Even so, after multiple discussions, Ryan expressed a willingness to follow up with an outpatient program and case manager. I was hoping these were steps towards building a meaningful life and that he wasn't appeasing me to secure his discharge. I suppose the hoping didn't matter in the end. Or did it? Was hope all that mattered when the patient gave up his and all I had left was mine for myself and those patients I wanted to help no matter what they did with their hope?

After multiple discussions with AD and with fellow colleagues, I started to realize that maybe keeping Ryan alive wasn't a realistic goal after all. Maybe it was not even my place to 'keep him alive' in any sense, behaviorally or otherwise. At this moment, I began to sense that I could not own his decisions or behaviors: he was not mine in any possessive sense at all. He was mine to be present to, to care for, and to help, but I saw I could not be responsible for him even if I willed it with all my might. His addiction was so advanced or 'end-stage.' We couldn't hospitalize indefinitely, especially when he was not expressing acute lethality. Yet his death made me question our decision to discharge him when we did. In some way, I felt responsible for his death. I also realized that while I was on the Palliative Care Service as a 4th year medical student, I did not feel responsible for a patient's death shortly after discharging them home or to hospice. Why would I feel more responsibility for discharging people with 'end-stage psychiatric illness' compared with those who have end-stage medical conditions? I believe that a dichotomy between 'psychiatric' and 'medical' illnesses continues to pervade our culture. Psychiatric illnesses are seen as deficiencies in behavior, character, or personality that should be remedied; therefore, they cannot be terminal. Somehow we believe they are qualitatively different from terminal cancer, diabetes, and pneumonia, maybe, in part, because we don't understand them as well.

As physicians, we accept death as a possible outcome of major illness. Unfortunately, it's an occupational hazard. Even with the best care, death can be unavoidable. Imagine that you are an emergency room physician treating a patient suffering from a heart attack. She is treated promptly, appropriately, and effectively; she improves. You feel like you saved her life, that the dangerous part is over. However, two days later, she has a fatal arrhythmia. You begin revisiting everything you did or did not do for her. But after determining you provided appropriate care, you might accept your limitations and confidently take care of your next patient. Why should suicide be different?

Just like we cannot fully control outcomes in advanced heart disease, we also cannot do so in advanced psychiatric illness. I strive to engage a patient with complete acceptance, unconditional regard, and without judgment, as have been modeled by my wonderful mentors. Sometimes a patient may be inspired to modify behavior in response. Other times, a patient may trust in pharmacological and behavioral interventions. In Ryan's case, I couldn't help him find another way to manage his social anxiety and opiate use disorders. He showed me my limits as a psychiatrist. This experience, along with the support I have received from caring mentors, liberates me from the fantasy of perfection and total control."

H. Patrick Driscoll, 2018

"Miller and Rollnick's book <u>Motivational Interviewing: Preparing People for Change</u> (2nd Ed.) was the most important book I read in my behavioral health training about how to be with others. It was that book that helped me see for the first time those 'unspecified elements of change' which for me is the stuff of any healing encounter. Because of that book, I could finally put into words what I had seen and dreamed of in working with my supervisor (and now colleague and co-author), Antoine.

I took the whole book all in, but what has stuck with me were a few elements that have since suffused my being with others. It was the active listening. I suddenly found out how much I had been talking, how much I had been missing, and how little I had been helping. I saw how little I had been validating others, which has since come to mean to me acknowledging the truth and value of another's experience. And I saw how much I had given into a sense of jadedness by not seeking out the basic sparks of hope and renewal in the chemistry that ought to exist between me and my patients, as it is in the best of motivational encounters. Specifically, I had been missing out on moments of evocation. MI has thus become for me the antidote to burnout and depletion. And this lesson is the one I yearn most to impart to any of the trainees I have been so blessed to work with.

One of the greatest moments of self-discovery occurred when I was an intern. AD was away from the unit, leaving me to lead a session with a patient with severe addiction and his shocked family. It was a patient I had been feeling so stuck about as had our whole team. I was so frustrated at my inability to engage with him and connect with what made him 'tick.' What I didn't know at the time was that I was missing getting his 'reasons for change.' And it was because I did not know how to ask him or listen!

What happened for me during the family meeting was as inadvertent as it was pivotal. As the family spoke naturally and spontaneously to the patient, I had no choice but to listen as they shared their painful concerns in the deepest and most poignant of ways. During what might be called a pregnant pause, I had a sense amidst the silence that something could be delivered. I asked the patient: 'What do you make of your sister's words? She said that she cries because she fears that she cares about you more than you might care about yourself, and she never wanted that for her little brother....' The patient who I feared had been feeling very guilty as the source of his family's pain began to cry as he shared that he never wanted to be the little brother who worried his family. It was a powerful identification he had made within himself that I know he and I had not connected about previously and likely would not have found between us. As I took in the family meeting in its aftermath, I thought about how uniquely the power of evocation can be harnessed in a family context as a reason for change in the identified patient. I loved the moment so much as I sensed within it a reconciliation of some of the conflicted parts within the patient as well as the healing of a critical fracture within the family. It was a decisive clinical moment that spurred me on to train further in working with families in a career in child and adolescent psychiatry.

My background in the addiction treatment of adults prepared me for the hardest challenges of working with young people, which often means helping adolescents with substance use problems. It was so difficult to help a vulnerable adolescent in a family context when his substance use behaviors were often not the cause but instead the consequence of problems within the family or beyond. It was hard to work with a family who the young patient needed so much but who was not yet prepared to look within itself to be part of the solution. It filled me with trepidation to approach the sensitive points within the family. It demanded of me levels of patience, tolerance, understanding, compassion, and empathy that I had not anticipated before choosing to work with this even more vulnerable population than the one I had learned to see in adults. I sought to bolster my capacities to do my best for the young people with addictions whom I saw on the inpatient adolescent unit by doing deep self-reflection, consulting with peers, and seeking supervision from my mentors. I sought to use for myself the same emotional regulation, distress tolerance, and mindfulness strategies that I was asking these young patients to use to manage themselves and their own urges. It was so hard to overcome within myself what was necessary to feel more gratified by this challenging work. I learned to reach within myself to not only treat the patient whose problems were sometimes nascent and not yet clearly defined, but to also engage the members of the family who did not always have a readiness to look within themselves for what to change or what to offer their struggling son or daughter.

Through working with these young patients and their families, I was humbled by how I often I underestimated the capacities within families to offer to their struggling children more than I initially judged. It hurt to be part of the moments when I felt I was less helpful than I could have been to a family because of my own frustrations or irritations. These moments occurred to me when I struggled to have the empathy and compassion that I have learned is so important to have to not just give better care but feel better about my work. But there were many good stories, too.

Sometimes a success was a matter of more attuned engagement with the parents to elicit the concerns that could frame an unspoken issue that they then all could confront together. Other times, the family succeeded for their young loved one despite my missing the mark after having reacted to my own prejudices and biases based on how I felt about a problem before I had gotten to know the most important facts available. The only way I could feel better and do better at my work meant acknowledging my shortcomings, mistakes, and limitations as well as claiming the painful feelings that went along with them. I had to change as a person by owning those feelings and working them through so that I could be freer to be more present (and helpful) to the patient. To be a better clinician in these exceptionally tough cases, I had to find a way to be honest with myself about how I could get in the way of therapeutic progress. I had once been so quick to point out what I assumed others had ignored, having first missed my blindest spots. These blind spots made it hard to see where to focus on the young patient and his family, and, because of these blind spots, I missed what I first needed to change in myself. It was through being able to recognize the motivational spirit in action from what I had seen through the examples of my best mentors that pointed me to an inward journey of inquiry and accountability for my own thoughts, feeling, and choices. It was only through this work on myself that I felt able to work with patients of all kinds (and ages) who I came to see as ultimately seeking to take responsibility for themselves and their lives. And as I saw it, this level of independence and self-responsibility was not possible for them as long as they depended on a substance to manage problems that they had not yet been able to do on their own. It was also a vision I had for them that I felt powerless to engage them about without first identifying a similar struggle within myself."

Conclusion

The process of engaging patients in transforming their lives has been the most inspiring work of my life, but I could not have done it alone. Ultimately, my teams of trainees inspired my growth as a person, by spurring me to challenge myself while simultaneously replenishing my spirit through our encounters together. I have wondered what it is about this shared clinical and educational dynamic that I have come to thrive on. On a daily basis, I have the opportunity to observe these trainees as they strive to integrate the motivational spirit in the deepest of ways, and I witness how this process changes them in ways so similar to the patients they care for. The students evolve as individuals in parallel to the very patients they are helping. Through this shared spirit, I see the trainees take responsibility for patient care, for building a caring relationship, and for their own clinical and personal growth. The trainees thus exemplify to me the very outcomes which they want for their patients: the trainees encounter within themselves those same internal resistances that their patients find to be the most difficult to surmount. In the best of cases, I am so gratified by the chance to facilitate the growth and development of a struggling patient. To be able to facilitate this development not just in patients but also in my trainees is to take in twice the rewards that I sought when I chose to work with this patient population to begin with. The trainees' reflections in this section are written so poignantly and candidly about how they bear witness to and care for their patients amidst struggle. I am inspired not only by their patients' journeys towards recovery but also by the paths that the trainees have chosen for themselves, both as practitioners and in life.

Recommended Readings

Cain DJ, Keenan K, Rubin S. Humanistic psychotherapies: handbook of research and practice. Washington, DC: American Psychological Association; 2016.

Douaihy A, Kelly TM, Gold MA. Motivational interviewing: a guide for medical trainees. New York: Oxford University Press; 2015.

Halpern J. From detached concern to empathy: humanizing medical practice. New York: Oxford University Press; 2001.

Kurtz E. In [Transcript of interview conducted by W. L. White]. Illinois Addiction Studies Archives: Normal, IL; 2008. http://www.tandfonline.com/doi/pdf/10.1080/07347324.2014.949123

Miller WR. Lovingkindness: realizing and practicing your true self. Eugene, OR: Cascade Books; 2017.

Miller WR, Rollnick S. Motivational interviewing: helping people change. 3rd ed. New York: Guilford Press; 2013.

Miller RW, Rollnick S. Motivational interviewing: preparing people for change. New York: Guilford Press; 2002.

Rosengren DB. Motivational interviewing skills: a practitioner's guide. 2nd ed. New York: Guilford Press; 2017. p. 179.

Schneider KJ, Pearson JF, Bugental JFT. The handbook of humanistic psychology: Leading edges in theory, research, and practice. Thousand Oaks, CA: Sage; 2001.

Epilogue

Values Shared and Values Learned

> "What am I myself? What have I done? I have collected and used everything that I have heard and observed. My work has been nourished by thousands of diverse individuals – ignorant and sage, genius and fool, infant and elderly. They all offer me their ability and their way of being. Often I have reaped the harvest that others have sown, my work is that of a collective being, and it carries the name of Goethe."
>
> —Goethe, from original conversation with Swiss scientist Frederick Soret, 1832

In this book, I wrote about how much I have been privileged to be witness to the complex experience of human suffering and recovery from addiction, and its impact on my clinical life. I explored how focusing on both humanism and science, and weaving them together defined my professional career. This integration is how I believe I can bring healing and guide the journey of "lovingkindness" [1] to those suffering from addiction. Offering personal reflections on building my identity as a patient-centered empathic healer was a challenging and unsettling task. Of course, through my own journey of self-discovery, I have accrued some common sense, compassion, humility, faith, hope, and, perhaps, wisdom. That is what I referred to early on in this book: *personal transformation*. I have always sought meaning, and through the journey of my career, working with people struggling to reclaim their lives, I found more than I would have imagined in unexpected places. My personal transformation started in centering my practice on listening with presence, empathy, and love. This perspective ignited a stronger sense of humility within me as I became more aware of my engagement with patients and the powerful impact of my interventions on their lives. The older and wiser I become, the more flexible and simple my approach to clinical work becomes. My slogan is as simple as the Serenity Prayer. As much as my empathy and compassion motivate me to invest in my patients the best I can, I have learned to balance it with a humbling awareness of the genuine limits of my helping abilities. Embracing and integrating mindfulness practice and the humanistic motivational interviewing spirit centered me and made me realize that my patients have the ultimate responsibility for changing themselves. The equanimity that I continue to cultivate in my clinical practice teaches me more about humility and frees me from the righting reflex.

In discussions about my career, a friend challenged me to identify openly my top values using the Values Card Sort as described earlier in this book. I have routinely incorporated this tool in my work with patients to help them identify 5–10 core values that are most central to their identity. So here they are, my top ten core values: compassion, flexibility, gratitude, genuineness, hope, humility, integrity, mindfulness, openness, and service. I also feel compelled to add "acceptance" as another core value. Exploring my values made me realize how much they match most of my patients' values. My practice is intertwined with my values. Respect, "creating relationships among equals," as articulated by Sarah Lawrence-Lightfoot in her book *Respect: An Exploration* [2], is central to my journey of "lovingkindness" in both my therapeutic work and personal life.

Thinking about acceptance and change, Carl Rogers pointed out the "curious paradox" that links the two:

> "When I accept myself as I am, then I change. I believe that I have learned this from my clients as well as within my own experience--that we cannot change, we cannot move away from what we are, until we thoroughly accept what we are. Then change seems to come about almost unnoticed." [3]

My patients, through my efforts in empathic listening and connectedness, have shared with me about their experiences. Their acceptance and appreciation of my helpfulness have made me more authentic and comfortable with who I am. After all the strategies and techniques are applied in my work with patients, I remind myself of my own flawed humanity as we collaborate, grieve, heal, and grow together.

Experiencing gratitude has shaped every therapeutic encounter of my career. My patients have given me the opportunity to help them to understand themselves, what and how they feel. For that I am filled with gratitude and I fully share it with them, hoping they will recognize and understand my genuine desire to help.

Reflecting on the most honest and transformative experiences in my career, Miller's writing in *Living As If: How Positive Faith Can Change your life* [4] enlightened me. It opened my eyes and my ears early on in my career when I needed faith to guide my professional and personal life. I have discovered and chosen *my* vision that helped me to understand my past, experience living my present, and plan my future. I have grown so much because of my patients, trainees, and mentors, who have inspired me to be who I am and at the same time strengthened my faith in myself and validated my path, values, and intention for my career. Only when doubt kicks in can I be reminded of my faith, not the faith of dogma and doctrine but the faith in "lovingkindness."

Kierkegaard [5] described hope as "a passion for what is possible" and the "hopeless" patient seeking treatment "hopefully" as doing so because of implicit hope. My value of hope has been inspired by my learning to strengthen and deepen connectedness, which for me is empathy in action. Throughout my therapeutic work, I learned that value by effortlessly learning to be patient, flexible, diligent, trustful, and confident. For me, it is hope that sustains emotional growth. Patients struggling with addiction come to me looking to restore their value system and meaning, to "Gather up the broken pieces that remain, that nothing is lost (John.6.12)." They put trust in me so together we gather all the fragmented, broken, disowned pieces of themselves and rebuild who they are. This is a mutual journey of healing and personal growth.

Reflecting on the unknowable and uncertainty in the science of practicing addiction as a healer, Anderson's statements [6] come to mind: the healer is no longer "a knower who is certain about what he or she knows (or thinks he or she knows)" but rather "a not-knower… and regards knowledge as evolving (p. 4)." Practitioners cannot and should not practice using *one size fits all*. Even with all theoretical paradigms and techniques considered and applied, it never captures the complexity of the unique experiences of suffering shared by patients and their families. I am a person blinded with misperceptions, who questions, disputes, wonders, struggles, suffers, and searches, just like *every* patient of mine. And I made mistakes. I misdiagnosed. I labeled. I judged. I disappointed. Personal therapy and active supervision and mentoring have strengthened my ability to be the effective healer I aspired to be.

In closing, I hope, dear reader, that in sharing my professional journey and personal growth, your practice working with persons with addiction becomes more mindful, enjoyable, rewarding, purposeful, and transformative. I can say with confidence that my addiction practice has made me a better patient-centered empathic healer *and* a better person.

References

1. Miller WR. Lovingkindness: realizing and practicing your true self. Eugene: OR; Cascade Books; 2017.
2. Lawrence-Lightfoot S. Respect, an exploration. Cambridge, MA: Perseus Books; 2000.
3. Rogers CR. On becoming a person: a therapist's view of psychotherapy, vol. 17. Boston: Houghton Mifflin Company; 1995.
4. Miller RW. Living as if, how positive faith can change your life. Philadelphia: The Westminster Press; 1985.
5. Kierkegaard S. The concept of dread (1844, translated by Lowrie W., 1957). Princeton University Press: Princeton; 1957.
6. Anderson H. Conversation, language, and possibilities: a postmodern approach to therapy. New York: Basic Books; 1997.

Index

A
Abuse, defined, 47
Acceptance and commitment therapy (ACT), 94
Accurate empathy, 5, 22, 56
　evidence-based practice, 21
　mindfulness approach, 22
　motivational interviewing, 21
Active case management strategies, 71
Active listening, 6, 7
Addiction, 36
　clinical practices, 60, 61
　effectiveness of treatment, 52
　history, 46–47
　motivational interviewing, 54–58
　pessimism, 47–51
　pharmacological treatments, 59, 60
　psychiatrist, 3, 36
　relapse prevention, 58, 59
　social stigma, 47–51
　theoretical models, 46, 47
　therapist effects, 53
　treatment, 39, 45
Addictive disorders, 45, 46, 48
　clinical observation skills, 5
　scientific and humanistic aspects, 4
Adolescent-like protagonist, 41
Against medical advice (AMA), 37, 38, 40
Alcohol addiction, 46
Alcoholics, 46, 48, 49, 53
Alcoholics anonymous (AA), 46, 80
Alcoholism, 46–49
　types, 46
Alcohol use, 25, 26
Alcohol use disorders, 35, 46, 52, 53, 59
American disease model, 48
American Psychiatric Association, 67
American Psychological Association Task Force, 21
Antidepressants, 12
Attentive/passive listening, 6

B
Behavioral health providers, 46
Behavioral therapy, 33
Berkson's fallacy, 61
Broken care relationship, 38

C
Case management, 33
Childhood stressors, 67
Christian morality, 47
Chronic medical illnesses, 36
Client-centered approach/counseling, 53, 54
Cocaine anonymous (CA), 81
Codependence hypothesis, 66
Cognitive-behavioral model, 59
Cognitive-behavioral therapy (CBT), 85, 94
Community reinforcement and family training (CRAFT), 67
Community reinforcement approach (CRA), 73
Compensatory self-control model, 48
Concerned significant others (CSOs), 65
Confrontational interventions, 51, 54
Co-occurring disorders, family members, 70–71
Counter-therapeutic approach, 39
Crystal meth anonymous (CMA), 81
Culture of addiction, 61

D

Depression, 11, 25, 26, 35, 36
Detoxification, 37, 57
Diagnosis unit, 16
Diagnostic and statistical manual of mental disorders (DSM)
  DSM-I, 46
  DSM-II, 46
  DSM-III, 47
  DSM-IV, 47
  DSM-V, 47
Diagnostic orphans, 47
Dialectical behavioral therapy (DBT), 94
Dichotomized approach, 52
Disease Concept of Alcoholism, 46
Disease model, 48, 50, 58
Disturbed family hypothesis, 66
Disturbed spouse hypothesis, 66
Drink-watchers, 81
Driving while intoxicated (DWI), 51
Drug addiction, 46
Drug dependence, 46
Drug rehabilitation programs, 35
Drug-related intoxication, 47
Drug use disorders, 61
DSM, *see* Diagnostic and Statistical Manual of Mental Disorders (DSM)

E

Egalitarian approach, 22
Empathic curiosity, 27
Empathic listening, 26
Empathy, defined, 53
Enlightenment model, 48
Episodic excessive drinking, 46
Evidence-based approaches, 21
  humanistic framework, 31
  objectivity, 32
  psychodynamic training, 31
  subjectivity, 32
  woolly-minded approach, 32
Evidence-based therapy relationships, 21

F

Families and addiction, myths, 66
Family-based interventions
  addiction treatment, 71
  clinical strategies, 71
  CRA, 73
  CRAFT, 72
  five –step approaches, 71
  treatment-related behaviors, 71
Feelings of loss, 40, 41

G

Gamblers anonymous (GA), 81
Gastro-intestinal bleeding, 24
Growth-fostering connection, 5

H

Habitual excessive drinking, 46
HARP, *see* High alcoholism recovery potential (HARP)
Healing, 3, 24
Healthcare practitioners, 4, 60
High alcoholism recovery potential (HARP), 53
Humanistic approach
  empathic connection, 98
  patient advocacy, 97
Humanistic practice
  self-discovery, 100–101
  treatment, trainee, 102–109
Humbling, 24

I

Interdisciplinary collaborative therapeutic approach, 33
Internalized supervision, 32, 35
Interpersonal determinants, 58
Intrapersonal determinants, 58

K

Kensho, 22

M

Medical school training, 6, 7
Medication-assisted treatments, 59
Mindfulness-oriented psychiatrist, 26
Mindfulness principles, 23
Moderation management (MM), 81
Moral model, 48, 49
Morbidity and Mortality conference, 15
Motivational engagement, 34
Motivational enhancement therapy (MET), 85
Motivational interviewing (MI), 21–23, 26–28, 54, 56, 57, 95–99, 101, 109
  accurate empathy, 56
  agape, 55
  client-centered counseling, 54
  defined, 22
  effectiveness of, 55
  healing love, 56
  humanistic approach

Index

empathic connection, 98–99
patient advocacy, 97–98
humanistic practice
  clinical, personal transformation, 95–96
  self-discovery, 101
  treatment, trainee, 109
inspired language, 26
OARS skills, 54
personal and clinical spirit, 99–100
substance use disorders, 55
treating addiction, 94–95
Multi-substance drug, 13
Mutual empathy, 26, 39
Mutual support programs (MSP), 83–89
  12-step programs
    myths, 83–84
    practical suggestions, 85
    reflections, clinical practice, 85–89
    12-step treatments, 84–85
  varieties of, 80–81

N

Narcotics anonymous (NA), 12, 81
NIDA Principles of Drug Treatment, 61
Non-alcoholics, 46
Non-authoritarian approach, 54
Non-HARP patients, 53

O

Opioid painkillers, 13
Opioid use disorder, 59

P

Parents' substance use, 67
Patient-doctor relationship, 12
Patient encounter, 3
Personality disorders, 47
Person-centered approach, treating chronic illness, 101–102
Person-centered MI-focused session, 40
Pharmacological interventions, 33
Pharmacotherapy
  addictive disorders, 60
  substance use disorders, 59
Polydrug use, 61
Polysubstance use, 37
Pray away addiction, 78
Project MATCH, 77
Pseudo-empathic skills, 26
Psychiatric disorders, 61
Psychiatry residency program, 3
Psychoactive substance abuse, 47

Psychoanalysis, 13
Psychodynamic training, 31
Psychotherapeutic approach, 5
Psychotherapy, 5

R

Relapse prevention (RP) theory, 58, 59
Relational-cultural therapy, 39
Research-to-treatment gap, 4
Robotic approach, 22

S

Screening, brief intervention, and referral to treatment (SBIRT), 60
Secular organizations for sobriety (SOS), 80
Self-listening skills, 21
Self-management and recovery training (SMART), 80
Self-medicating depression, 13
Skepticism, 4, 46
Skid row alcoholics, 78
Spirituality and religion
  beliefs and tradition, 78
  healthcare practitioners, addiction, 79–80
  treatments, for addiction, 78–79
Suboxone®, 40
Substance abuse, 47
Substance dependence, 47
Substance use disorders, 3, 4, 47, 50, 52, 53, 55, 58–61
  family and children
    family settings, motivational engagement, 70
    toxic environment, 67
    traumatic experiences, neighborhood, 68
Substance use treatment system, 60
Supervision, defined, 32

T

Therapeutic listening, 12
Therapeutic skills, 22
Therapeutic techniques, 23
Thich Nhat Hanh's Zen Buddhist philosophy, 23
Total laryngectomy, 33
12-step programs
  myths, 83
  practical suggestions, 85
  reflections, clinical practice, 85
  12-step treatments, 84

U
U.S. temperance movement, 46

V
Vicarious introspection, 5
Vipassana, 79
Virtual free association, 38

W
War on drugs, 46
Withdrawal symptoms, 14
Women for Sobriety, 81

Z
Zen Buddhism, 22
Zen listening, 26
Zen mind, beginner's mind, 31
   Zen philosophy, 22

The manufacturer's authorised representative in the EU is Springer Nature Customer Service Centre GmbH, Europaplatz 3, 69115 Heidelberg, Germany. If you have any concerns regarding our products, please contact ProductSafety@springernature.com

Printed and bound by CPI Group (UK) Ltd, Croydon, CR0 4YY

23/03/2026

02076399-0002